In *Growing Older*, Gary Kindley offers our generation a reflective gift about what aging gracefully means in an era in which people imagine they can opt out of growing older. Perhaps a little more intuitive insight and a little less Botox is the order of the day. This book is a mature alternative to chemicals!

—David Mosser, Ph.D.
Senior Pastor, First United Methodist Church, Arlington TX
Adjunct Professor of Homiletics—
Perkins School of Theology
Southern Methodist University, Dallas, TX

Dr. Kindley shares with us keen insight and gentle wisdom on the Fear of Aging which has profound implications for our future well-being on the individual, familial and societal levels. We avoid thinking about what we fear. Whether it's our own health, our retirement finances or the future of Medicare and Social Security, avoiding the topics of aging will not be a successful strategy. Thank you Dr. Kindley for naming the fear and giving us help and hope in facing it.

—Chris G Spence
President, Wesleyan Homes
Past Chair Texas Association of Homes
and Services for the Aging

Growing Older Without Fear [is] a book that will inspire and help those facing their senior years without trepidation...[Dr. Kindley's] national survey on aging will be a resource for whoever wants to face the future with enthusiasm and optimism....
—Mayor Tom Leppert
City of Dallas, TX

Gary Kindley's writing is clear, honest and makes this book a pleasure to read. I was deeply moved by the wisdom of these pages. I believe that many of the leaders with whom I have worked through the years will find it one of the best!
—Bill Evans, CEO
The Evans Group

GROWING OLDER

WITHOUT FEAR

For Jim & Cheryl:

Joy, peace, and

Courage for the journey!

Mary Lindley

GARY G. KINDLEY

GROWING OLDER
WITHOUT FEAR

the nine qualities of successful aging

TATE PUBLISHING & *Enterprises*

Published by Tate Publishing & Enterprises, LLC
127 E. Trade Center Terrace | Mustang, Oklahoma 73064 USA
1.888.361.9473 | www.tatepublishing.com

Tate Publishing is committed to excellence in the publishing industry. The company reflects the philosophy established by the founders, based on Psalm 68:11,
"The Lord gave the word and great was the company of those who published it."

Book design copyright © 2010 by Tate Publishing, LLC. All rights reserved.
Cover design by Amber Gulilat
Interior design by Nathan Harmony

Published in the United States of America

ISBN: 978-1-61663-290-8
1. Self Help: Aging
2. Health and Fitness: Healthy Living
10.04.21

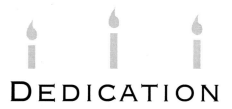

DEDICATION

For my father, Eldon Kindley, whose lessons about life and aging were lived each day, with details shared over lunch each Friday at Luby's Cafeteria.

For my sister, Judy Kindley Pacatte, whose gifts as a teacher and care-giver continue to bless so many lives on their journey.

For David, John, Jeff, Kristen, Alex and sons and daughters everywhere, to give you some tips about what is ahead. Remember the "honor your father and mother" commandment (and buy long-term care insurance).

ACKNOWLEDGMENT

This book is in response to my own questions and anxiety about aging. I have both laughed at and believed in the maxim, "Growing old is mandatory; growing up is optional." It has taken me just over half a century to arrive at this point of my own journey, and it will likely be several more decades before I see congruence between growing up and growing old!

I am a Baby Boomer, born at the end of 1955, just twenty-eight days after Rosa Parks refused to give up her seat to a white passenger while riding on a Montgomery, Alabama, city bus. Perhaps that was a foreshadowing of my own journey, as my Caucasian, East Texas mother and Caucasian, West Texas father raised my sister, Judy, and I in an integrated neighborhood in southeast Fort Worth, Texas, that began to shift from predominately Caucasian to a predominately African-American population as I entered high school. This unlikely pairing taught us what it meant to be a good neighbor, and in doing so, also modeled tolerance, acceptance, generosity, kindness, love, justice, service, and faith (with some appropriate righteous indignation thrown in for good measure).

There are many people who helped make this project possible. My first round of gratitude goes to those who have assisted with travel and/or lodging as a part of this process: John and Danya Reider, Betty Ralls, Claude and Anita Nelson, Jake and Linda Jacobson, Garth and Molly Heggenes, Wes Wheeler, Bob and Billie Tuttle, Glenna Fairman, Shorty and Mildred Jenkins, Gene and Jan Bingham, and Woody and Beverly Thompson.

I am tremendously grateful for the editorial assistance of two wonderful people. Beth Battles, Ph.D., Chairs the English Department of Texas Wesleyan University and took time from her sabbatical to read and edit my manuscript. Roanne Harless, a gifted educator and grammar guru, provided invaluable insight while reading and re-reading, and was willing to accept late-night telephoned questions about syntax and usage. I was also aided by the very helpful input of Sylvia Morrison and Myrna Maas, whose spiritual intelligence, wide-eyed perspective, and delightful humor made the project more fun. Kelvin Meyers, a forensic genealogist and researcher, offered both feedback and assistance with bibliographic research. I am also grateful for Ted Beneski, who tutored me in statistics so that I might tabulate and apply the survey appropriately.

I have been blessed by the congregation of First United Methodist Church of Colleyville, who granted sabbatical time to help me bring conclusion to this book. It was also a blessing to receive the many nudging inquiries, "When is it going to be published?" as a means of encouraging my follow-through.

Others whose names must be included for their support, whether they offered wise counsel, encouraging words, supportive prayer, caring calls, or house-sitting during my time away: Mary Bassett, Doug and Ellen Boston, Phyllis Brandon, John and Monica Burks, Bishop Ben Chamness, Carl Chelette, Janice Chelette, Reverend Dr. Jerry Chism, Stella Davis, Ramiro and Renee DeLaGarza, Reverend B. Connally Dugger, Bill Evans, Dominick Farinella, Lt. Gen. (Retired) Carl and Edith Franklin, Reverend Jay Fraze, Reverend Dr. Larry George, Lisa and Jeff Glass, Reverend Milton Guttierrez, Reverend Gary A. Lindley, Bishop Michael Lowry, Malcom Maas, Reverend Dr. Tim McLemore, Errol Miller, John and Trish Norman, Ed and Ruth Olson, Melissa Omernik, John and Diane Pace, Edward Cleveland Payne III, Melanie Riggins, Stephen and Ashley Riggins, Reverend Kent Seuser, Bob and Betty Straub, Reverend Ed Volfe, Reverend Bob and Mary Weathers, Reverend Lara Whitley, and Barbara and Randy Wilson.

Throughout my journey, but especially in recent years, I am most grateful for the encouragement of two mentors and friends: Reverend Jack Scott, Ph.D., and Reverend T. Michael Young, D.Min. Jack and Mike understand the importance of asking probing questions when others want simplistic answers, seeing the opportunity in what most would call obstacles, and offering grace when it is least expected.

Speaking of questions, this preface wouldn't be complete without expressing profound appreciation for the many people who were willing to be interviewed or to participate in the survey on aging and fear. Your courage to respond and to express your individual concerns, joys, anxieties, and expectations made possible the pages that follow.

Live long. Be well. Love much.

—Gary G. Kindley
Dallas, Texas
January 2010

TABLE OF CONTENTS

AN IMPORTANT
INTRODUCTION

(So don't skip to Chapter 1!)

I would like to believe that life is a journey over which we have a great deal of control; though I know that is not entirely true. I am quite certain that life is about choices (wise and poor), as well as experiences (good and bad). I am also certain, as human experience bears witness, that life's journey is not unlike a deep and flowing river. The river of life flows as it will, with human choices as well as random events causing their own ripples in life's current.

Water has the power to change things, both giving life and taking it away. Water's surge can bring breath-taking beauty or cause devastating destruction. The flow of life's river also changes us. Whether we go-with-the-flow or try to fight the current, we are still mortal beings. Our mortality is characterized by a truth that we cannot ignore: our physical selves change as we age.

There are things that we can do about the changes that

occur to us and our bodies. We can take action to be healthy, and to even retard the effects of aging, but aging nonetheless marches on. It seems that the rational response to those parts of our journey that are immutable is to determine how we will respond to them. If we know that aging is a part of life, then our attitude toward such inevitability determines how we enjoy the ride. Our attitude makes all the difference in whether we go with the flow or attempt to change the current.

From my perspective, life is also a bit like the tram that shuttles you between the parking lot and the main gate at *Six Flags* amusement park. We can try to outrun the tram (which my friends and I did in our youth), or we can jump onboard and enjoy the ride with the refreshing breeze blowing through our hair. The tram can take us through the exhilaration of the roller coaster and then return us to the mundane routine of a ride in the family car, but the tram runs its course whether we choose to get on it or not.

I mentioned the idea that our lives are also impacted by an element of randomness. Such randomness in life is not to say that life is without purpose, but we need not approach life with the set-in-stone, double-predestination philosophy expressed by John Calvin (1509–1564). God has infused our world with serendipity and chance along with certainty and purpose. Perhaps it is a component of free will, but nonetheless, some stuff just happens, and it need not all happen for a specific reason beyond the serendipity of life.

Given all that, this book is about perspective and attitude on life as a whole and on our own life specifically. It is about how we see life, ourselves, and what happens to us as we grow older. It is a witness to the perspectives of people of various age, ethnicity, geography, and spirituality. This book is about the wonder of life that is worth embracing rather than fearing, relishing rather than escaping.

Time marches on and gives us choices. We can learn the cadence and march along, or hear a different drummer and keep a different pace. We can follow the main road with its unexpected detours and see where it takes us, or create new paths for others to follow. We can also pretend that there is no parade and miss all of the fun!

Personally, I want to enjoy the ride. I choose to believe that the thrilling times will overcome the challenging ones whether or not they outnumber them. I am grateful and encouraged to learn that there are many who believe as I do. May we learn from each other and from our own journey. Most of all, may we enjoy the experience and cherish the ride!

The Divine, Higher Power, and God

There will be some who are uncomfortable with this book because they want to explore the relationship between growing older and fear, but they are not comfortable with spiritual or religious language. This is not a religious book as some may define it, but it is a book that addresses the spiritual component of life. If this bothers some who pick up this text, then the words from the Alcoholics Anonymous "Big Book" may serve you well: "take what you like and leave the rest." There is likely something helpful here for anyone who wishes to find it.

Working as often as I do with people who have been abused by religion or those in recovery from addictions, I strive to focus on spirituality rather than a particular set of doctrinal beliefs. This is especially necessary as clients begin to rebuild their faith around loving acceptance rather than judgmental condemnation. Though my personal spiritual beliefs are anchored in the teachings of Jesus and I identify myself as Christian, I consider my tolerance of people from other faiths or those with no belief in a transcendent being to be a gift and not a weakness or dilution of my beliefs. This may trouble those who express very strongly-held religious beliefs and confuse tolerance with a lack of conviction.

In this book you will see the capitalized words "God" or "Creator" used as the proper noun that most of us are familiar with in the Judeo-Christian tradition. This is typically what I use in my personal thoughts and prayers. You will also see the word "Divine," representing the transcendent and used interchangeably with "Higher Power" or "God," though I have found that the term "Divine" carries a more universal meaning. "Higher Power" is commonly used in Twelve-Step Programs in order to accommodate those who are seeking recovery from some addiction and who may come from a religious or spiritual background that uses other names for "God." These persons may also be struggling to accept that there is a transcendent quality of life, and so "Higher Power" is a better choice when referring to transcendence in the most general sense. Do not be confused when finding all of these terms used in this book, just keep in mind that a reference to "Divine gifts" can mean the same thing as "gifts given to us by God" or qualities that are transcendent in nature or origin.

Using the Reflection Questions

This book is designed to be used individually or as a part of a study group or class. At the end of each chapter, you will find a set of questions entitled, "For Reflection." If you are reading this apart from a group, reflect upon these questions for your life. You may wish to journal your reflections or responses.

If you are a participating in a study group, book club, or class, use these questions as a part of group or small group discussion. Some individual reflection questions are so rich with possibilities that more than one session could be spent "unpacking" the deeper meanings or ideas that these questions can evoke. Enjoy the discussion and do not be afraid to share your own experiences, feelings, and thoughts, even if you have a contrarian viewpoint; that is what gives life's journey depth and richness. There may be someone who has been waiting their whole life to hear your story in order to better understand their own.

Above all, embrace and relish this opportunity to examine the perspective that you bring to life and ways you might make your journey more meaningful, joyful, and productive. This is your life, your chance, your ride, your today, and your tomorrow. Ready. Set. Go!

ON THE RUN

The Predator and the Prey

"Some say that time is a predator, always stalking you—but I have come to feel that time is a companion, accompanying you along the journey. Time reminds you to cherish every moment, because they may never come again."
—Patrick Stewart as Captain Jean Luc Picard
Star Trek Generations[1]

"Fear is our greatest enemy."
—Winston Churchill

"I don't buy green bananas any more."
—Eighty-seven-year-old grandmother on aging

Body, Soul, and Solace

From science fiction writing, to twentieth-century history, to the sage wit of a wise woman, these words help to center our thoughts when we consider the nature of human life, our sacred journey, and our mortal fear. Fear, like aging, is an elusive thing that we can allow to misdirect us from what is truly important—living!

What only startles one—the faint scurry of a mouse across a shiny wooden floor—evokes panic in another. One of the oldest and most familiar stories known to the world, the Genesis story of the Bible, taps the nearly universal fear of venomous serpents to manifest the Satan, the evil one who tempts Eve and Adam from their pristine state of grace.

Fear can be paralyzing or motivating. Fear can cripple us from living or propel us forward into life-saving action. The fight-or-flight response identified by behavioral psychologists can turn ordinary soldiers into heroes. That rush of adrenaline as our endocrine system responds to fear has enabled one-hundred-fifty-pound mothers to lift heavy objects off of their injured child or firefighters to accomplish superhuman feats to save a fallen comrade.

Fear is not limited to the extraordinary. Fear can be found in the ordinary, everyday human interactions in the home, school, or workplace. The power and influence of personality can cause a spouse to tremble in fear before an abusive partner whom they are afraid to leave, a child to walk two blocks in pouring rain to avoid a school bully, or an employee to endure humiliation and injustice at the hands of a domineering boss for fear of losing their job. Fear is real; it is both universal and unique to each human being. What about the fear of growing older?

Growing older is a process that is both natural and inevitable. At issue is the *fear* that we attach to aging. The fact that aging is, of itself, ancient is an irony that offers little comfort or satisfaction—as if aging was a persona whom we could annoy with its own mortality. It has been a process that has eluded understanding, control, and evasion. It has been a naturally occurring progression that has taken place since the origin of life, with hope of immortality limited to the realm of the Divine. Hence ancient cultures such as the Egyptians, Babylonians, Greeks, and Romans gave their gods and goddesses the properties of immortality, or associated them with issues of life and death. Human vulnerability, our own mortality, required help from those whose powers exceeded meager human limitations. It was the changes of aging from which vulnerable mortals sought transcendent help in order to avoid the inevitable trek of human mortality.

The Changes of Aging

We all age in both body and mind. We all face the normal changes that come from mortality. For some, the loss of beauty is the most overwhelming and debilitating loss to imagine. Grief is found in the inevitable sagging of our skin, wrinkling of our face, and vanishing pigmentation as our hair begins to gray. For others, it is the loss of physical abilities. The weekend warrior, who once-upon-a-time could paint the house following the morning five-mile jog, discovers that muscles tire more quickly and that distance seems more formidable.

Others are less fearful of changes with their body than with changes in their relationships. What if they outlive their family? What if they outlive their friends? What if there is no one left to care for them as they grow older?

Still others are concerned with the material and business matters of life. Will they have sufficient financial resources to provide for themselves, their spouse, and/or loved ones as life progresses? Will they be able to remain in their home as they grow older or will they need to move to a place for assisted living—a retirement or nursing facility? Will they be able to afford such a place? Will all of their estate be used up so that they have nothing to leave their children as a legacy?

There is the common fear of losing our mental abilities. Memory fades and our cognitive powers are not as quick as they once were. With medical advancement comes longevity, and with longevity comes the increasing likelihood of developing significant cognitive impairment, dementia, or Alzheimer's disease. Those over eighty years of age have a 50% chance of developing dementia or Alzheimer's in their lifetime.[2]

Definitions and Starting Points

It is important to distinguish between the fear of growing *older* and growing *old*. Our frequent dread of the process of aging is the focus of this book. Growing old implies a particular defining threshold that, once reached, declares that you are now old! There is no such universal point, though individuals may associate certain milestones or indicators as the defining mark between growing older and having grown old.

Defining marks of growing old are, of course, a matter of one's perspective. For children, anyone as old as their parents— or if they are generous, their grandparents—are considered old. For teenagers or young adults, it may be a similar definition, or a decade demarcation such as thirty or forty. For many adults, the age of fifty, sixty, or retirement, defines "old age." Still others use not only a criterion of longevity, but also of ability. Someone may be deemed old when physical or mental abilities begin to fail, or fall to an ill-defined point of dysfunction.

My focus is directed toward how different people perceive and approach growing older. This also includes the ways we can learn to boldly embrace the process and nature of our maturity rather than crumble in the face of the inevitable course of human mortality. For the purpose of this book, I use the following definition:

Human aging is the naturally-occurring process and associated experience of diminishing physical and mental abilities, youthful appearance and vigor over a period of time.

If this defines aging for our purposes, then what defines successful aging? As Tom Kirkwood, a Professor of Biological Gerontology at the University of Manchester, put it, "The challenge is to age as successfully as we can."[3] What is the criterion of successful aging? What makes one person's experience better than that of another?

Can you "fail" at growing older? If so, do you get "mulligans" or "do-overs," or is aging simply graded "on the curve?" If you don't do well the first time, do you get to take the course again, or is that only if you are a believer in reincarnation? Does money determine success, as in how much of it you have to afford retirement and nursing home residency? Does good health determine successful aging, and if so, if I need to take medication to survive, am I a partial failure?

Americans are an especially competitive lot and it is of no surprise that many live as if successful aging is a category for competition. Considering this perspective, against whom would this competition be held? Are we competing against each other, poor health, bad luck, or is this a grander competition about mortality—the realm of death and God?

If this is a competition, then who are the judges? When things do not have the outcome we desire, how and where do we appeal our circumstances? Do we blame our physicians, sue drug companies, point fingers at government, or take countless societies' historic fallback position: blame it all on God? Perhaps the issue is not about competition or blame, but about control.

It is not the process of growing older that is the focus of some, but how much control they have over it. As long as some people feel "in control" of life, then they would define that as successful aging. When the truth is realized—that life, health, finances, and relationships can never be completely controlled by them—it can be a depressing, anxiety-provoking shock. Perhaps that is why so many people "put up a fight" when it comes to the process of aging.

Medical science offers us a framework to put successful aging into perspective. According to an article published in *Clinical Geriatrics*, a journal for gerontologists and gerontology-related health-care professionals, successful aging is based on three identifying components:

1. Low risk of disease,

2. A high level of mental and physical functioning, and

3. An active engagement with life.[4]

Whatever our definition of aging, successful or otherwise, consider to what lengths we will go in an attempt to stop—or at least significantly slow down—this process.

Evidence of a Fight

One has only to visit a local pharmacy to get a glimpse of the amount of money American consumers spend on cosmetics and beauty treatments. To put this in perspective, one company, *Avon Products*, who historically has not sold their beauty products through retail pharmacies or stores, showed a market value of $22 billion dollars in 2004, and twice the market value of General Motors in 2008 (before GM's market value declined as the automotive giant faced bankruptcy). This, from a company whose wares you typically do not see at the store, is clearly remarkable. Can you imagine the value of all of the many other cosmetic and beauty market corporations? These are the corporations whose ubiquitous products are seen on the shelves of stores of most every variety, and are the focus of ads in magazines and newspapers, and on billboards and buses. [5]

According to the American Society of Aesthetic Plastic Surgery, in 2007, Americans spent in excess of $13 billion for cosmetic surgery; $8.3 billion was spent on surgical cosmetic procedures, and $4.7 billion went to non-surgical cosmetic procedures. From 1997 to 2007, the number of cosmetic procedures increased 457%. On average, 47% of all cosmetic procedures are performed on people ages thirty-five to fifty, with liposuction and Botox injections the most common procedures requested. The typical liposuction procedure to remove fat from areas such as the hips and abdomen averages about $3,500 per procedure.[6]

Botox injections to *temporarily* remove wrinkles (heavy emphasis on the word *temporarily*), the most commonly requested non-surgical aesthetic procedure, has grown in popularity with the number of procedures increasing an average of 37% per year. Most patients spend about $1,000 for the treatment, with many repeating the injections more than once over a period of two years.[7]

If all of this isn't enough of an indicator of our collective "fight" against aging, consider one more revealing statistic. *Nielsen Media Research* reported that 10.1 million television viewers watched the season finale of ABC's *Extreme Makeover*.[8]

What does this say about us? When fear of growing older becomes so self-centered and self-consuming that we choose to spend on *temporary* wrinkle reduction the same amount it would take to feed a child in a third-world nation for *two years*, we have a serious priority deficit.

Cosmetic procedures can transform birth defects into natural beauty, improve scarring from trauma, and even slow down the process of aging when it appears more rampant in some than in others. But there comes a time when we must ask ourselves when enough is enough. What are we fleeing? What are we trying to regain? Why? What would it take for us to embrace the natural flow of life and the person whom we are and shall yet become in mind, spirit, *and* body?

The process of growing older is, for some, a predator that is stalking and we are the prey. For them, there is a sense of panic when some arbitrary, self-determined time in life is reached and they realize that what was their youth of yesterday will not be again. For those who are wise, it is also a time to look to the wisdom and maturity that tomorrow holds. It is a time to appreciate that there is wholeness and well-being yet to be realized and celebrated. Moments in time, both behind us and yet-to-come, are meant to be cherished, not dreaded. Each new day brings new possibilities.

How is it for you? Is time a predator or a companion? Where do you stand?

Is aging:

- something from which you are running?
- a process you are tolerating?

- a part of life you are denying?
- a reality you are accepting?
- a mystery you are exploring?
- a journey you are making?
- a ride you are taking?
- a challenge you are facing?
- an opportunity you are embracing?

For Reflection

1. What is one pre-conceived idea about aging that you have that you may need to reconsider?

2. What do you consider to be "successful aging?" Is there a "tipping point" when our efforts to age gracefully by means of health and beauty products and aesthetic (plastic) surgery become more frantic efforts to avoid our own mortality?

3. Do you think that our mortality helps us to better cherish others? Do you think that the reason some people do not cherish life is because of their understanding—or lack of understanding—of their own mortality?

NAMING OUR FEAR

From What Are We Running?

"So, first of all, let me assert my firm belief that the only thing we have to fear is fear itself..."
—Franklin Delano Roosevelt

"If you fear change, leave it here."
—Business writer, Rhonda Abrams,
reporting a handwritten note she once saw over a tip jar

"It's not that I'm afraid to die, I just don't want to be there when it happens."
—Woody Allen

Taking It All for Granted

Americans are aging into a longevity that has been increasing since 1900. One news report explains it this way:

This [increase in life expectancy] is the result of several factors, from the most basic—improvements in public water treatment and sanitation systems—to remarkable advances in medicine and health care. Certain types of unhealthy behavior, such as smoking, have steadily declined due to effective public health education.[9]

Of course, the ever-increasing taxes, euphemistically named "sin taxes," added to tobacco by federal and state government have likely had some influence as well. In 1900, one of the leading causes of death among children was simple diarrhea.[10] Acute illnesses and communicable disease were leading causes of death compared to chronic illness today, such as cancer, heart disease, and stroke.[11] Could it be that this ongoing rise in life expectancy—this delaying of our death—is contributing to a false belief that we can somehow outrun our mortality?

If that is true, this next fact will be a wake-up call for the baby-boomer generation: due to obesity and hypertension (high blood pressure), at least half of Americans ages fifty-five to sixty-four are in worse physical health than those born a decade earlier when they were the same age.[12]

Perhaps we have taken the longevity rise for granted. Maybe we are relying too much on advances in medicine and health-care to keep us alive and healthy beyond reasonable expectations. It is easier to take a pill than to spend thirty minutes on a treadmill three times each week, and so we hold-out for quick-fix medical advances, hoping for research to find that Cheese-whiz and Fried Oreos are surprisingly good for us! Science has its limits, and there is no pharmaceutical substitute for eating a balanced diet, regular participation in aerobic activity, and adequate rest and sleep. Still, we are a people who are anxious, if not outright afraid of growing older, and our anxiety and fear are pervasive, though varied, across the human experience.

Fear of the unknown is usually why people don't take a first step. Some go boldly, most do not. The questions, excuses, complaints, and rationalization that we put forth in order to avoid facing life's realities reflect our own resistance or even paranoia about ourselves and our future. We avoid or ignore that which we are afraid to face, and use evasive words, attitudes, and behaviors that ultimately lead ourselves astray.

We rationalize:

- I'm not growing older; I'm not retired yet!
- Why should I put so much effort into exercising when they'll invent a pill in a few years to fix whatever is wrong with me?
- I'm not sick, so why should I worry about trying to stay well?
- It takes time to eat healthy, and I'm too busy!
- I'll change to a healthier lifestyle when my business slows down!
- I'll change to a healthier lifestyle when my kids are older!

We also act irrationally, worrying about that which is not important at the expense of that which is truly vital. We take action and make choices based on irrational thinking:

- If I don't do something about my wrinkles, what will others think of me?
- If I am not beautiful on the outside, then I am not beautiful!
- It's worth whatever it costs to stay looking young!
- If I can't stay young-looking then there's no need to keep going!

We "awfulize" or "catastrophize" and think in terms of all-or-nothing when things aren't as we might hope. "If I don't have (pick one or more):

- larger breasts
- slimmer thighs
- more hair
- less hair
- shinier hair
- longer hair
- bigger muscles
- hairy chest
- smaller nose
- less fat
- less gray
- bigger penis
- longer nails
- bigger lips
- thinner eyebrows
- thicker lashes
- nicer skin
- whiter teeth
- or _____

then it is awful and I am not good looking!"

We spend billions of dollars on superficial beauty while three billion people on this planet live on less than two dollars per day.[13] Worrying about that which is not important at the expense of that which is truly vital—human life—can be considered immoral and reflects the narcissism, indifference, and/or ignorance of affluent societies.

Believing In Ourselves

Our self-esteem is the root of so much of our attitude, choices, and behavior. Rather than accept ourselves for who we are, we may strive to be something or someone whom we are not and never shall be. It is noble to strive for self-improvement and growth in body, mind, and spirit. It is unhealthy to deny ourselves the self-acceptance that is so vital to being the whole person that God made us to be. We are made as a part of God's wonderful gift of creation, and there is blessing in accepting ourselves for who we are. No human body is perfect, and the adage is true that "beauty is often in the eye of the beholder," but a strong confidence in ourselves and our potential is a healthy response to life.

What is our fear? From what are we running? Perhaps we are trying to run from our own shadow or our own self-doubt. I have experienced greater self-confidence and a life-embracing outlook in persons with physical and mental disabilities than in many who have no genuine reason to complain about their circumstances. Personally, I consider the following truth a key idea to remember:

> *What we believe about ourselves and the extent to which we accept ourselves foreshadows the outcome of our life's journey.*

When we choose to integrate the natural ebb and flow of life into our reality, when we stop rationalizing and start realizing, when turmoil and anxiety turns to trust and acceptance, we stop running from our own shadow and being chased by the fears of our own creation. It is at these points of awareness that we begin to live in the present moment and be comfortable in our own skin. Sadly, fear is a place where many tend to dwell and the human experience includes times when we are fearful of life and the process of mortality.

To better understand our fear of growing older, I began by surveying adults aged eighteen and above who lived in the United States and asked them if they had anxiety or fear about growing older. I soon learned to remove from the survey population anyone under the age of thirty. Most people age eighteen through twenty-nine seemed to have no point of reference regarding my questions. Though they had concern about beauty and looks—as cosmetic sales can attest—they had given little, if any, thought to aging. They still held a feeling of pseudo-immortality. Persons in this age group tend to think that growing old is a long, long way off. Basically, the idea of growing older—or fearing aging—seemed out of their realm of understanding.

My survey was not exhaustive, nor did it sample large populations of every ethnic group in the United States, but it was a sufficiently random sampling to serve as a valid reflection of the thoughts, feelings, and fears of many Americans. I interviewed hundreds of people who were Anglo, Hispanic/Latino, African-American, Native American, Asian or Pacific Islander. I surveyed an affluent area where the median income was greater than $175,000 to determine if financial wealth affected one's perspective on growing old; it did. Several surveys were conducted through churches and synagogues in order to assure the inclusion of a spiritual perspective, while other surveys were conducted with "person on the street" interviews in different regions of the country to get a broader section of the population. These included Muslims, Buddhists, Native American spiritualists and other spiritual expressions, as well as the viewpoint of persons who identified themselves as agnostic or atheistic.

I spoke with people in restaurants, bars, health clubs, shops, spas, airports, subways, casinos, hotels, businesses, hospitals, nursing homes and retirement homes, as well as at conventions, service clubs, Chamber of Commerce meetings, and various events. I interviewed people in person or by written or e-mailed surveys in Washington, California, Nevada, Colorado, New Mexico, Texas, Oklahoma, Missouri, Illinois, Iowa, New York, Pennsylvania, Washington, D.C., Florida, Louisiana (post-Katrina/Rita storms), and Tennessee. I included urban dwellers and small-town residents. Participants were business owners, laborers—both white-collar and blue-collar employees—executives, homemakers, students, the retired, and the homeless. I visited with persons who were unemployed and looking for work, and also with many others who were employed, full-time or part-time, and either happy with their career or looking for something better.

What People Report about Growing Older

When I asked people age thirty and above if they had any anxiety or fear of growing older, ninety percent of those surveyed said yes. The ten percent who said that they had no anxiety or fear about growing older were spread evenly across age groups from ages thirty-five to sixty-nine. In other words, 100% of those interviewed age thirty to thirty-four, and age seventy plus reported anxiety or fear about growing older. One person in the seventy-five to seventy-nine age range responded "some fear" but did not list any specific fears.

I next asked them to list their greatest fears about growing older. These five responses below became a recurring theme in the surveys or interviews. Whether one or more fears were listed, these were the five most commonly reported.

- Deteriorating physical abilities—including the loss of vigor and strength and the inability to do the activities or daily tasks that they enjoy or take for granted.

- Deteriorating mental abilities—including impaired memory (98% of responders expressed memory concerns), loss of concentration, dementia, or other cognitive disease.

- Loneliness—the increased possibility of losing spouses, partners, friends, and other loved ones who are currently a source of significance, security, companionship, and comfort.

- Loss of youthful appearance—bearing the normal progression of aging, including the graying or loss of hair, loss of muscle tone, loss of skin tone, loss or gain of body fat, and wrinkles.

- Financial instability—the uncertainty of financial security due to outliving one's resources, insufficient lifetime income, or a lack of planning, skill, knowledge or market stability.

In addition to the five greatest areas of concern listed above, other areas of concern, fear, or loss regarding aging (not ranked) included:

- The changing relationship between parents and their adult children, including caring for and "parenting" one's aging parents, or feeling "parented" and controlled by one's adult children.

- The feeling of disappointment, grief, or defeat from not accomplishing one's life goals.

- Fear of failure, whether personally or professionally.

- The realization of life's folly—that we are not in control, nor can we be—juxtaposed to the youthful view of "I can do anything" or "I am bulletproof."

- Being "passed over" in one's career by more youthful and less-experienced co-workers.

- The changing relationship between parents and teenagers/young adults as the innocence of childhood naturally moves to the defiance of adolescence and the independence of young adulthood (Interestingly, this was only reported by young mothers).

- Never finding a lifetime spouse or partner.

- Allowing one's fears to limit possibilities of success or progress.

- Never seeing one's sports team win the Pennant/Cup/Super Bowl (you might surmise which gender humorously included this).

- Fear of how one might die.

- Fear of a dreaded disease.

- Fear of the process of aging and how it might unfold.

- Concern of having no care-giver as physical or mental self-sufficiency decreases.

- Fear of pain.

- Fear of rejection, loss of respect, or a tarnished legacy should one's life secrets be made known before or after death (I surmise that this includes crimes, indiscretions, or flaws of character or ethics).

- Worry about of the afterlife.

- Fear of salvation/damnation for one's self, loved ones, and/or friends.
- Concern of having never found one's purpose, destiny, or path.
- Fear of irrelevance—not making a difference in one's lifetime.
- Fear of the unknown, of one's uncertain future or destiny.
- Grief of never having had children.
- Fear of being unable to have children.
- Grief of the end of a family business.
- Grief of being the last in one's family tree.

While my interview subjects were racially diverse, one or more of these fears were generally reflected across lines of race, class, and most cultures; though their importance and intensity varied person-to-person.

Concern over loss of physical ability and mental ability were statistically even. Surprisingly for me, loss of financial resources was of greater concern than loneliness for many of the more affluent responders. Loss of financial resources was a concern for many across socio-economic lines, but the more affluent, the greater the concern. For the general population, with average to upper-middle-class incomes, loneliness was a slightly greater concern than loss of youthful appearance.

It is important to note that the affluent people who I interviewed, some of whom were quite wealthy, were what I would characterize as the "working wealthy." Some had made their own fortune and had risen from low or middle-class incomes. These were generally not independently wealthy folk for whom money was of no concern. It is quite possible that loss of financial resources was worrisome due to a fear of being unable to sustain the level of living to which they had grown accustomed. This would be especially true should physical or mental aging impede them. Still, there were some whose wealth seemed their greatest concern despite having more than adequate finances to live quite the luxurious lifestyle and provide for themselves and their spouse/partner.

There was one group of people I interviewed whose culture had a much different perspective of aging. Fear of growing older was minimal because they looked at it from a more positive and accepting perspective. These were Native Americans, and from them we can learn a great deal.

For Reflection

1. What is your greatest fear about aging? What factors influence your concern?

2. Are your fears or concerns driving any actions that you are taking?

3. How do your relationships, spirituality, and financial situation impact your concerns about aging?

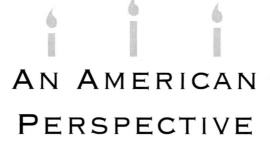

AN AMERICAN PERSPECTIVE

Native Americans and the Journey of Life and Aging

"Everything on the earth has a purpose, every disease an herb to cure it, and every person a mission. This is the Indian theory of existence."
—Mourning Dove Salish (1888–1936)

"I have seen that in any great undertaking it is not enough for a man to depend simply upon himself."
—Lone Man (Isna-la-wica), Teton Sioux

"I love to roam over the prairies. There I feel free and happy, but when we settle down, we grow pale and die."
—Santana, Kiowa Chief

Refreshing Conversations

I had a wonderful experience interviewing Native Americans during visits to New Mexico and Oklahoma. I had already received some written survey responses from Native Americans earlier in the information-gathering phase of this project. At this point, I had not drawn any conclusions regarding how Native American culture viewed growing older. I did not anticipate any significant difference in viewpoint than that of any other ethnic group surveyed. My interviews were no different than ones I had done in any of the other places I had visited. What was different was the recurring theme of the responses I received.

As I strolled the winding, narrow streets and large central square of Santa Fe, I spoke with a diversity of people whom I passed along the way. Some were talented craftsmen and craftswomen, their wares and artistry beautifully displayed at the famous artisan market outside the Governor's Palace. Some were locals dining in one of the many popular restaurants, or travelers who had come from other regions of the country or the world to sample southwestern cuisine. Others were shoppers in boutiques, galleries, or one of the many eccentric stores that bring a tourist flavor to this centuries-old city.

I gave to each what had become my standard spiel. I told them that I was writing a book about aging and wanted their perspective. From my earliest interviews as I began this project, I learned through experience that people were more likely to talk with you if you told them that what they said might get published in a book. Most people tend to be wary when stopped by a passerby for conversation. I discovered that when they have an idea where the conversation is headed and that there is a chance that they might find their words in print and on the shelf at their local bookstore, their interest peaks and they lower their defenses, becoming less guarded and remarkably candid.

Whomever I spoke with got the oral version of the same written survey that so many others had completed by now:

1. "Do you have any anxiety or fear about growing old?"

2. "What would be your greatest fear?"

3. "What other fears do you have about growing old?"

At this point I would inquire about their coping skills by saying:

People who tend to cope well with aging may have one or more of these characteristics in their life. How important are these to you, ranking them from one to four?

> _____*A plan of self-care*—choosing to lead a healthy life through adequate nutrition, exercise, medical care, and awareness of health issues

> _____*An attitude of optimism*—keeping a positive outlook that views life from a larger perspective and considers aging as a normal process of one's journey

> _____*A spiritual perspective*—believing in a spiritual, transcendent component of life and cultivating one's spirituality just as one would care for their physical body

> _____*A focus on the well-being of others*—focusing outward toward the well-being of others, seeking to be of service to others rather than dwelling on one's own difficulties

Over the course of the interviews and surveys, it became obvious that the four areas that I listed as coping skills were too limiting. I had initially articulated these four to identify the most frequently evident healthy coping skills I observed. In order to have some consistency in the survey, I had offered them for participants to rank while also allowing them to choose another coping skill that was important for them.

These "Other" categories developed a pattern of their own,

requiring that I expand and rework my list of identified healthy coping skills from four to nine. People who age most successfully tend to:

1. Claim a sense of well-being

2. Maintain a grasp of stewardship

3. Choose to focus on others' needs

4. Keep an attitude of optimism

5. Enjoy a sense of humor

6. Nurture a spiritual perspective

7. Make a plan of self-care

8. Develop a supportive network

9. Hold a vision for the future

I will say more about each of these coping methods in another chapter, but the Native American people with whom I spoke tended to speak of the importance of many of these areas more frequently than did anyone else. Most were not satisfied to add only one item to the "Other" option of the survey's question three.

A consistent pattern emerged from these many interviews with Native Americans of most every age, from thirty to eighty-plus. For Native American culture, aging is a part of the journey of life and is nothing to fear. Here are some of their perspectives.

Anthony, age fifty, construction worker:

> I never thought about *[growing older]*. I don't worry about it. For Native Americans it is a part of life. Thirty, forty, fifty are no big deal. They are just numbers. Life is life—

days go on. I'm getting some pains—my shoulder bothers me now, but that's all just a part of it.

You grow to appreciate family more and more. What I think about is enjoying my children and grand children growing up.

Anthony on death:

Black people and white people are upset over war. *[At the time of this interview, the United States was occupying Iraq with no plan of withdrawal, and President Bush's approval ratings were plummeting.]* They are protesting losing their sons and daughters. I have two members of my family who are *[serving with the military]* in Iraq, my niece and nephew. That's life, too. For Native Americans, war and fighting have always been a part of our culture. We have always struggled.

Joe, age sixty, artisan:

I am coming up on, let's see—I guess this will be sixty *[years]* for me this year. I have an eight-year-old son—my youngest. I served in Viet Nam, a Marine Assault Group. The V.A. *[Veterans Administration]* has helped me educate and care for my family. Now, I sell my jewelry. It is my gift, made with my own hands with my mark on the back.

You gain wisdom with your gray hair. Culture is important, and remembering who you are is important. Many of these people *[he refers to other Native American artisans around him]*, they forget their culture. They don't even dance anymore *[tribal dancing]*. My tribe, we dance—we keep the culture. That is important, to remember who you are. I still live on the reservation. We have a dirt road—no pavement—in front of my house. That is who I am.

Joe, on fear of aging:

> I don't fear getting older, but if I had to pick one thing that might bother me it would be my body—my physical ability. This body has seen me through life. I work with my hands. I've never been afraid of work. I wouldn't want to lose that *[ability]*.

Michelle, age thirty, artisan:

> I don't have any fears about growing older. I don't worry about it. If I had to choose one thing that may worry me at all, it would be finances. I make a living here selling my jewelry. If I wasn't able to do that, I don't know what that would mean.

I asked Michelle whom she thought was the most fearful of growing older, men or women. Without a moment's pause she said, emphatically, "Women!" followed by laughter. Michelle is an urban resident who does not reside on a reservation. Still, her response was very similar to that of Anthony and Joe who have much more life experience.

Lilly, age eighty-one, retired (Lilly was gambling in a casino on a reservation)

> My health is not what it used to be, and I know that it's not going to get any better. That's just how it is. I go on. I am strong. That's life. I have my family and my friends and that's enough.

Harry, age seventy-five, retired. Harry was alternating between the sauna and cold plunge at an outdoor spa. He did this, with quiet reflection, for more than an hour during my visit—outlasting all of the younger men there that day in this modern version of a "sweat lodge."

This *[growing older]* is life. There is nothing to talk about.

It was a great blessing to speak with Native Americans and hear their cultural perspective that seemed almost universal—growing older is simply a part of the journey of life. There is no need to worry or fear, for life shall unfold as it will. No amount of worry will slow it down or change it, but only make one dread the moments that lie ahead and fear the unknown still to come.

The Native American perspective is a liberating one. If they were not a people who embraced life, I would say that it is almost a passive outlook. It is not passive, for being passive implies no intention or action. There is preparation and work taking place here. There is saving financially, living actively, embracing lovingly, and remembering joyfully. There is intentionality in preserving culture, embracing the past, and being open to the future. There is living life by being an active participant, not a passive bystander, while not resisting nor struggling with the certainties of the journey, such as growing older. Our Native American brothers and sisters have much to teach us of growing older, and we have much that we need to learn in order that all might embrace life to its fullest potential.

How We Die or How We Live?

There are other ethnic cultures, as well as individuals within a category of race or ethnicity, whose ethnic, cultural, religious, or familial customs or obligations give them a unique approach to aging. Two examples are found in the Korean and Japanese cultures. The Korean culture commonly sees aging parents moving in with one of their adult children. This reflects the Korean cultural respect for the aged and honoring parents. Though they are not the only ethnic culture to do this, it appears far more normative than in some others, who typically resist having their freedom and privacy compromised by the presence of a dependent parent. For some Korean families, this move may also happen at an earlier age than is typical so that parents' financial needs are taken care of by an affluent son or daughter. This may be done both out of an attitude of respect and of pride for their ability to do so.

Long-standing Japanese cultural perspectives of personal responsibility and self-reliance, combined with longevity due to medical advances, have led to an increased incidence of suicide among the elderly Japanese population in order to avoid being a burden upon their adult children or others. This sort of thinking is troubling, and not confined solely to Japanese culture. The phenomenon has not gone unnoticed by the Japanese electronic industry. In order to allow continued independence for older people requiring additional assistance with their daily routine, companies are now offering robots that serve as household assistants. The robots replace the need to rely upon human assistance and help to alleviate some older adults' sense of burden on their children while allowing them independence and enjoyment of their lives.[14]

Other individuals of various races and ethnic origin demonstrate an approach to living, aging and dying that serves as a healthy and vibrant role model. Perhaps they are influenced by the admonition of their religious tradition to honor father and mother. Perhaps they have learned the lesson, taught by parents or grandparents, that it is good and right to care about others throughout their life. Their enthusiasm and human kindness reveal how good life can be when it is cherished and shared.

Betty Ralls is a good friend of mine who knows how to have fun in life. Though she lives in Texas, she has a mountain home in Colorado that she has generously shared with friends through the years. She has the gracious gift of hospitality and entertains all of her guests with the elegance of a most thoughtful and benevolent hostess. She celebrates life through the way that she cherishes friendships, laughter, family, loyalty and faith. You might say that these qualities are in her DNA, for when her father died she described him well when she said, "He died living!" Betty has experienced many of the same struggles that come with life's journey, including the loss of a husband whose death came far too soon. Still, it is her attitude and spirit that carries her forward and draws her friends close.

People like Betty, who live life as a celebration, draw others to them like a magnet. They choose to focus on living rather than worry about dying. They are often positive, enthusiastic people whose energy is stimulating and whose outlook is contagious. Even so, attitude or outlook alone cannot determine all outcomes. As investment companies are required by law to say: "Past performance is not a guarantee of future results." We can be leisurely floating down the river of life and not know that a precipitous waterfall awaits us around the bend.

Though we cannot necessarily determine the future or ultimate conclusion of our life, we still explore questions out of our natural—if somewhat morbid—curiosity. One commonly considered question is: "If you could choose how you die, would you?" No one desires to die of dread disease or make the deteriorating slide toward dementia. For some, it is not only the fear of growing older, but the fear of what aging could bring that evokes the greatest fear.

Many years ago, I counseled with a man whose mother had

a rare disorder that resulted in premature and severe cognitive deterioration. Genetic testing was able to determine that, though his children escaped the genetic flaw, he did not. How does one prepare for such inevitability? He knew that he would lose his mental faculties. He knew that the well-educated man whom he had become (he held a PhD in chemistry) would deteriorate to someone unable to recognize family or care for himself. His wife and sons knew that—far before his time—he would decline to a point necessitating round-the-clock care while his peers played golf and enjoyed their grandchildren. In the years that followed, that is exactly what happened.

His decline was gradual rather than precipitous, but the eventuality that we all knew was inevitable could not be stopped. His illness gave him insight as to how his life would unfold—more awareness than many of us might know, or want to know, about our future. He and his family accepted it as a part of their life's story. If they had been given no advance warning of his developing impairment, would his life have unfolded differently? Perhaps knowing what was ahead gave him awareness to cherish each moment with family and friends.

Some individuals with such desperate prospects for their future might seek to take their life, but such a choice also carries its own cruelties and heartbreak. Both suicide and euthanasia remain culturally taboo, as well as illegal in Texas and most everywhere, while also being mired in a firestorm of ethical, social, and religious concerns. His faith, and the faith of his family, would not consider such a choice. Instead, he chose to live out his days—his story. He, his wife and their family are some of the bravest people I have ever known.

Growing older has genuine concerns, and to deny that it does would be to diminish the reality of our mortality. We are not in complete control of the journey, and there are sometimes detours that we would rather not take. To acknowledge this and then relinquish anxiety about that which we cannot change is a positive, healthy step toward growing older without fear.

If we view life as a highway rather than a river, even in the scary twists and hair-pin turns of the road, it is helpful to remember that God is at work for good along the way. Like most of the major highways in my home state of Texas, it seems that the road of life is always under construction. When navigating pot-holes that crews are diligently working to repair, one is reminded that smooth, uninterrupted thoroughfares are infrequent or hard to find. Cancer, dementia, and other dread disease can become formidable roadblocks or at least hazardous detours with uncertain headings. There are circumstances when we cannot choose how we might face death, but we can choose how we will face life. Some people live their life dying, and others die while still living. It is not how we die but how we live that most defines us.

Successful Aging

In the first chapter, I referred to a three-point definition of successful aging as outlined in an article from *Clinical Geriatrics*:

- Low risk of disease
- A high level of mental and physical functioning
- An active engagement with life.[15]

It is clear that actively engaging life includes not resisting the normal flow of life. This is not to say that accepting the normal flow of life includes the passive acceptance of disease or that which could be prudently changed for the better.

Active engagement includes putting up a fight against that which robs us of wholeness physically, emotionally, interpersonally, and spiritually. We may be in the river of life, but we need not drown if we can swim! By nutrition or medication, we actively work to fend off the damaging effects of diabetes, Alzheimer's, or any number of maladies that might afflict us. We seek medical treatment—conventional or alternative—to stave off cancer or other ailments that diminish the joy of life. When we struggle with relationships, seeking the wise counsel of those with greater knowledge and experience helps us to work through conflict and difficulty. Through actively engaging life and health, we diminish our disease—our dis-ease—and maintain as high a level as possible of mental and physical ability.

Such is successful aging. Such is successful living: embracing, loving, growing, accepting, working and caring about life and those who share the journey. These are just some of the qualities of people who age well and graciously. Let's next consider how they do it and what we all can do to age with success and style.

For Reflection

1. How do you define successful aging? How does your definition address any fears about aging you may have?

2. Do you believe that your definition of successful aging would be any different based on your age (do you think that it would change from age thirty to fifty to eighty)?

3. Do you agree with the predominant Native American perspective that aging is a part of life? What role, if any, does faith and spirituality play in your view on aging?

TAKING A DEEP BREATH

Coping Strategies That Work

"The secret to staying young is to live honestly, eat slowly, and lie about your age."

—Lucille Ball

"Life is short. Marriage is long. Drink up, it will make it go faster."

—Shirley MacClaine as Katharine Richelieu,
the cynical and irreverent grandmother
from the movie: *Rumor Has It*[6]

"Good health is simply the slowest way a human can die."

—anonymous quote on a calendar
in the office of gerontologist Dr. Paul Kim

Coping Characteristics

There is a wide variety of philosophies and approaches, many of which are quite hilarious, that people express when the conversation turns to growing older. Let's consider again the qualities most common among people who cope well with the challenges of life and aging. Those who are less fearful about growing older, who strive to live in the present moment and not to dwell on yesterday or be fretful about tomorrow, demonstrate several of these characteristics in their life. They:

1. Claim the gift of well-being

2. Maintain a grasp of stewardship

3. Choose to focus on others' needs

4. Keep an attitude of optimism

5. Enjoy a sense of humor

6. Nurture a spiritual perspective

7. Make a plan of self-care

8. Develop a supportive network

9. Hold a vision for the future

The more of these qualities you possess, the more likely you are to cope well with growing older. Some of these characteristics may, at first glance, appear to be quite similar. A closer look reveals that each has its own distinctive quality, making it a vital component of living well and aging with grace and peace.

I have grouped these nine qualities into three subcategories that I call *Principles*, *Perspective*, and *Plan*. These three groupings help us to understand why each of these characteristics matter and why randomly picking a quality is not a path toward successful aging.

Principles are values to which we anchor ourselves, grounding our being in these ideals. The three Principles of healthy aging are:

- Claim the gift of well-being
- Maintain a grasp of stewardship
- Choose to focus on others' needs

When I look at these three Principles, I think of them as centered in the "I am worth it" values of self-esteem and self-worth. To better understand how self-esteem and self-worth tie together the Principles of successful aging, consider the observations of Dr. Ron Lorimar and Dr. B. Glenn Wilkerson. As a result of their work with the ARKGroup (formerly the Children's Center for Self-Esteem, Inc.) they differentiate self-esteem and self-worth in this way:

> Self-esteem is created in an affirming, nurturing environment characterized by unconditional love (i.e., where a person is loved and accepted for who he *is* rather than for what he *does*). Self-worth is a person's concept of self, based on a sense of personal competency. Self-worth links performance with feelings of worth and emphasizes achieving and *doing*.[17]

When we, through healthy self-esteem, accept that we are worthy to claim the gift of well-being (we accept ourselves as the sacred beings that we *are*), we treat our life, our world and our relationships as sacred by acts of stewardship and service (focusing on the needs of the world and others). Our fulfillment—our sense of self-worth—comes by living out our Principles (self-worth through what we *do*).

Perspective is an outlook, a world-view that perceives and responds to what happens on the journey from a particular viewpoint. Three key Perspectives of healthy aging are:

- Keep an attitude of optimism
- Enjoy a sense of humor
- Nurture a spiritual perspective

If Principles are the heart of our values, then Perspective is the lens through which we look at the world. We choose our viewpoint, though life-experience and our formative environment as children and youth can have a great impact on that choice. Optimism, humor and spirituality help us to see life differently. They can exist in even the most oppressive circumstances, like the bright yellow flower that bursts forth from the crack of a concrete slab. There were prisoners of Nazi death camps who never lost hope, surviving to inspire the world and generations to come. They refused to surrender their faith, hope and humor in the most somber of circumstances, though their situation gave them every reason to despair and surrender.

Optimism and humor give us a better look at life, and nurturing a spiritual perspective helps us see a completely unique dimension of life. Some find developing a spiritual perspective to be the most difficult challenge they can undertake. Many persons in twelve-step addiction recovery programs stumble over steps one and two: believing in a power greater than themselves to help them, and surrendering their unmanageable lives over to this Higher Power/God. Ultimately, spirituality is about relationships—both with God and with each other. A spiritual perspective sees life as a spiritual journey, or a journey of spiritual people, and recognizes the transcendent.

Finally, is our *Plan*; it is our action-plan and the route we have chosen for our journey. It is how we get from birth to death to life. The three vital components of a Plan for healthy aging are:

- Make a plan of self-care
- Develop a supportive network
- Hold a vision for the future

Plan is distinctive from Perspective, for it is neither a viewpoint nor an attitude. It results from the integration of our Principles and Perspective. We cannot make a plan of self-care without starting with our Principles and choosing to see ourselves as worthy and our tasks as a sacred trust. It is difficult to develop a supportive network if we don't feel good enough about ourselves to reach out and make friends, or if we remain so self-centered that we do not listen to or care about others. Our vision for the future is greatly influenced by our Perspective, whether optimistic or pessimistic, spiritual or earth-bound. Holding a vision for the future is not merely about viewpoint as much as it is about destination. Vision considers where we are headed—what is our ultimate goal.

How we take care of ourselves and go about developing a supportive network may change. In my case, I ran on my neighborhood streets when I was thirty and use the elliptical trainer and treadmill at my gym now that I am in my fifties. This is my new approach to self-care, because it is easier on my joints and muscles. As a university student or a church pastor, I had an automatic support network of peers or parish members. Now, as a counselor and writer, I must be more intentional about participating in groups, classes, and social organizations while maintaining my relationships with longtime friends.

The vision we hold for our future also varies with time. We may have both short-term and long-term goals. Our vision may look days ahead, years ahead, or to the end of our life.

We may ask ourselves what we want to accomplish as our ultimate mission in life and this may be one specific goal such as, to be rich. Our mission might also be one over-arching theme such as, to be happy, that spans our various objectives throughout life. Whether a "bucket list" of accomplishments and experiences we went to check-off before we "check-out," or an ultimate purpose—to make a difference—our vision is an opportunity to put our life in perspective.

Though in the pages that follow I have numbered these qualities for easy reference and divided them into the three subcategories, this should not be interpreted as ranking them in order of priority. They are too complex to be simply ranked. It would be misleading to do so, for ranking can imply that one is more important or that they should be addressed in a particular order.

Having these Principles, Perspective and a Plan are all vitally important. It is not necessary to decide which comes first, for they are ingredients that you blend together in the recipe that is uniquely your life. Your journey is your own, and you do have a choice as to which ingredients you will seek to include and how much you desire to add to the mix. For you, one may be the "icing on the cake" that makes your life the most delicious. Each life has its own unique flavor. Some people settle for bland, others have robust taste, and there are those who like life spicy!

Let's now consider these three essential groupings of ingredients that can anchor our life for a healthier journey. In this chapter, we will look at the first group, the three defining *Principles* of successful aging.

Claim the Gift of Well-Being

What does it mean to "claim the gift of well-being?" It sounds like well-being comes packaged in a brightly wrapped box awaiting us to tug at its satin ribbon (Note to men: If you prefer, substitute "cardboard" for "brightly wrapped" and "rope" for "satin ribbon" to make this a more rugged, masculine metaphor). If so, where do we find it, must we buy it, or do we already have a "claim check" and it is waiting to be picked up? Do we inherently know what it is to be well, or is well-being akin to spirituality and it is more a matter of individual perspective and one's own experiences? Is wellness in our DNA and that is why some families have a history of longevity? Could it be that well-being is an inherited pattern of behavior and interests that makes some families more athletic, more earth-friendly, more laid-back, or more at peace with themselves and those around them than are others? Is it ego or discipline that compels some to work diligently to keep their bodies strong and healthy, while others view physical fitness with apathy or disdain?

A friend of mine recently underwent a cardiac stress test following an episode of chest pain while climbing a flight of stairs. His physician told him that there was no sign of heart disease; he was simply out-of-shape. Several weeks later I inquired if he had been getting any exercise. He said, "I'm too busy and my chest doesn't hurt anymore!" My friend is a better example of being in denial than claiming the gift of well-being!

Clearly, wellness is not solely a matter of individual perspective, for there is irrefutable scientific evidence of how genetics, as well as our choices and behaviors, play a role in the physical health of our bodies. Having the viewpoint that cigarettes do not cause ill health, or that excessive consumption of alcoholic beverages is healthy does not alter overwhelming and undeniable medical evidence to the contrary.

The gift of well-being represents what life is meant to be—a journey of experiences that are rooted in both divine and human relationships. *How* life goes is different for everyone and is affected by countless factors, including choices and chance, chromosomes and circumstances, faith and futility. Well-being exists when we embrace, nourish, and integrate the physical, intellectual, emotional and spiritual components of our life into our experience. To put it in terms of the transcendent—where well-being is ultimately rooted—the human lifespan is a spiritual journey and corporeal existence that consists of physical, intellectual, emotional and spiritual experiences. All of these are necessary for us to be complete. To be truly well is to be whole, and though it is not the same for everyone, two universal constants of wholeness are to *accept* and to *integrate* who we are into our life experience and claim our self-esteem (value) and self-worth (purpose).

Physical, mental, emotional, or spiritual difficulties or physical or mental deformities need not limit our well-being when we integrate our unique nature into our identity. If we believe that Creation is a gift of God, then we are both recipients of the gift as well as bearers of that gift. Like any gift, we can accept it, reject it, ignore it, or neglect it, but even if we deny it the gift is still there. The truth of God's love and existence is not dependent upon our acceptance of that reality. In contrast, claiming the gift of well-being requires that we embrace the transcendent nature of life, for we are never whole apart from the Divine. We are people of body, mind, *and spirit*, and a three-legged table with only two legs is broken and collapses under its own weight.

Eleanor Roosevelt, the late widow of President Franklin D. Roosevelt, is often cited as the source of this bit of wisdom: "Yesterday is history, tomorrow is mystery, and today is a gift; that is why we call it the present." Successful aging involves living in the present moment, something that many people rarely do. When we live in "the now," this present and precious moment, we claim the gift of well-being that is offered to us—regardless of our present circumstance—every moment of every day.

Eckhart Tolle, philosopher and spiritual teacher, emphasizes living in the present as crucial to being fulfilled and our whole true selves. I think often of his simple but profound story that is a lesson in letting go of yesterday to live in today:

> The inability or rather unwillingness of the human mind to let go of the past is beautifully illustrated in the story of two Zen monks, Tanzan and Ekido, who were walking along a country road that had become extremely muddy after heavy rains. Near a village, they came upon a young woman who was trying to cross the road, but the mud was so deep it would have ruined the silk kimono she was wearing. Tanzan at once picked her up and carried her to the other side.
>
> The monks walked on in silence. Five hours later, as they were approaching the lodging temple, Ekido couldn't restrain himself any longer. "Why did you carry that girl across the road?" he asked. "We monks are not supposed to do things like that."
>
> "I put the girl down hours ago," said Tanzan. "Are you still carrying her?"[18]

Living from our true center—finding contentment by living in the present, rather than the past or the future—is to grasp the nature of well-being and claim the gift of wholeness essential for successful living and aging. This explains why people can claim and live the gift of well-being, though external circumstances might lead others to perceive them as someone who is not at all well. Some of the most centered and whole people I have ever met lived with physical challenges that would overwhelm many of us. Congenital impairment that leaves bodies without limbs, vision, and/or hearing imposes seemingly insurmountable hardship, yet cannot stifle the resilient human spirit of many who rise above such ongoing obstacles. Such inspiring and amazing people do not focus on their limitations, but claim the gift of well-being that comes from within.

One of the saddest things we do to ourselves and others is to use overly-simplistic thinking and myopic tunnel vision to define an image of what constitutes being "gifted." We miss the larger picture and true depth of the human experience. A Divine gift can be any of the innumerable qualities, skills, natural abilities, intellectual capacity, or physical, emotional or mental aptitude that each individual brings to life. We may dismiss the Divine gifts that lie within each of us because we are seeking the superficial values of human shallowness: "good looks" and financial wealth.

By some standards, Albert Einstein was a failure at relationships, inconsistent academically, and troubled emotionally as he struggled with depression. Einstein could have chosen to focus on his failures, doubts and disappointments, and never worked to develop his gift of grasping mathematical and theoretical concepts that eluded others. Nick Vujicic was born without arms or legs, but this amazing young man travels the world sharing his inspirational story with millions. His theme says it all: "From No Limbs to No Limits!" His positive, enthusiastic outlook, given his considerable, life-long physical limitations, makes the typical woes that most of us have appear petty.[19] Well-being is the essence of claiming the gift of God that lies within each of us—our unique identity and birthright—and living from our true center.

Consider the Book of Beginnings, or what we know as Genesis, the first book of the Bible and one of the most ancient documents ever written. It is a part of Torah and a creation story with relevance across Judaism, Christianity, and Islam, even bearing kinship to the creation stories of other ancient cultures. It tells us that the primary nature of the Divine is that of Creator. God made everything that we know, from dark to light, stars to planets, water to land, animals to humans, and God saw that it all was *very* good! At creation, well-being was to live in a state of harmony and grace with all that is; God, people, and planet. Such harmony is still a worthy objective, however impossible it is to attain.

As each generation grows and matures, we can choose to advance beyond childish bickering and tribal warfare and to successfully evolve into a people of harmony and grace. If not us, who? If not now, when? If we believe that such a state can never exist, then it will not, for we will not strive to make it so. True wholeness is akin to the tenet of eighteenth century theologian, John Wesley, whose idea of "going on to perfection" speaks to being made complete in our divine humanity. To begin to understand Wesley's concept, it is important to realize that he is not speaking of "perfectionism," which is an unhealthy and compulsive cycle of human thought and behavior—expecting one's self and others to never make a mistake. Wesley, an Anglican cleric who is considered the father of today's Methodist Church, urged all who believed in Christ to aim for perfection, a wholeness in mind and spirit that Wesley described as "true and holy living," and "having the mind of Christ." Wesley never denied our humanity and imperfection of thought and deed. He described Christian perfection as something that we may never quite attain, while still being a desire for which we strive. Wesley, a rabid reader, prolific author, gifted thinker (he first associated what we define as depression with dysfunctional electrical patterns in the brain), social reformer, ecumenical leader, and preacher to throngs of avid listeners, was a faithful visionary and man of the people, not some esoteric dreamer.[20]

Though some may perceive this as a fanciful construct with no grounding in daily practice, striving for wholeness is a daily choice and intention. It is a way of living, grounded in the principle that harmony with self, others, creation, and Creator is a greater good. To carry Wesley's teachings a bit further, Wesley's general rules were simply: Do no harm; do good; love God. These rules may be simple in language, but they have extensive consequences for deed, word, and spirit.[21]

To claim a sense of well-being is to be content in one's circumstance, seeing life as an evolving part of a larger journey. Contentment is not apathy nor being a victim and failing to work to improve your life, but to be content in the moment of whatever your life circumstance might be. Not the same as optimism—though most who are content with their well-being are optimistic—a sense of well-being is a state of contentment that holds firm in spite of changing health or circumstance. Well-being is separate and distinct from good health, as illustrated through the amazing lives of physically challenged folks who live in a state of contentment though their bodies may not be as healthy as others. To put it another way, someone can live in a state of well-being and not be physically well.

Well-being means to keep a sense of balance, a distinctive

intention to strive for peace and harmony within one's own self and the world around you. It is to focus on wholeness in body, mind, and spirit. Well-being permeates actions and attitudes, diet and determination, to live in a state of contentment while striving for greater wellness.

In a matter of six months, five pastors whom I knew died of heart attacks. The youngest was in his fifties. All were sudden and unexpected deaths of men who had focused so much time on the care of others that they often neglected their own well-being. Some were optimists, but that is separate from having a state of well-being that moves one's life toward wholeness in both deed and desire. Thus, thought and action toward self and others must work together to accomplish wellness. A sense of well-being recognizes the need to live as a whole person, not compartmentalized or focusing only on body, service, self, or spirit. Wholeness is intentional.

Some years following the deaths of those five clergy, a physician conducted a survey of clergy in the same region to discern their state of wellness. Following the five deaths, the local United Methodist hospital system had offered low-cost health club benefits to pastors and their families. A no-to-low-cost counseling program was put in place to address issues of stress and relationship difficulties. In spite of these and other efforts, the state of clergy health and clergy attitudes of well-being had made little change.

It wasn't that the clergy lacked the resources to improve their life; they lacked a sense of well-being. A genuine sense of well-being is not content with self-neglect and an apathetic lifestyle. A genuine sense of well-being seeks to live in wholeness and celebrates both life and health as a precious and divine gift. A genuine sense of well-being does not dwell on one's own problems, but neither ignores self-care. A genuine sense of well-being does not require the approval of others to live one's life to the fullest, nor does it demand that others live their lives in a certain way in order to be accepted. Genuine well-being sees life, health, spirituality, and relationships as integral components of wholeness—what it means to be a whole person of God—and proceeds to act in word, deed, attitude, and spirit to bring all of these vital elements into harmony.

Maintain a Grasp of Stewardship

Stewardship has historically been associated with management (such as the chief steward of a household in the Roman era), or servanthood (the room steward on your cruise). Stewardship also has religious connotations; various faith traditions talk about being stewards of life. Stewardship may be one of the most difficult concepts to grasp if humanity's own typical lack of stewardship is an indicator. For example, consider one global aspect of stewardship, the environment of the planet.

In the area of environmental stewardship alone, humankind has had a bleak if not abysmal track record. Were you to cling to the position that climate changes are merely a routine of nature's evolution rather than evidence of the theory of human-caused "global warming," you would still be hardpressed to deny that human industrial activity has had a devastating impact on our planet. Stripped forests, polluted water, oil-stained coastlands, extinct and endangered species all testify that we have not helped our planet to "age gracefully." To use a different metaphor, we have gone beyond "spending our children's inheritance" in our gluttony of earth's resources, to leaving future generations destitute of an environment that can sustain life and lifestyle as we know it today. Our children cannot replace species that are vanishing on "our watch," nor can future generations create habitat, rainforests, or clean wells for drinking water if our actions today make it impossible.

To best understand the meaning of stewardship for our life, we turn to one who is likely the most powerful voice for stewardship in history. Not just environmental or financial stewardship, but stewardship of all that life is about. Listen to the radical teachings of Jesus, and stewardship takes on a much deeper and significant meaning. I find it significant that the New Testament records Jesus talking about stewardship so often that, were a pastor to address the subject in a weekly sermon, almost every third Sunday would be a lesson on stewardship! There are numerous stories about what is genuine treasure (love, relationships, God's way of just and peaceful living), what need be our true priority (not things), and the importance of not letting possessions be held too close while allowing people to be kept too distant.

Jesus taught:

- Relationships are priceless and sacred gifts (Matthew 5:23–24).
- Giving is to be done with humility (Matthew 6:2–3).
- Be on guard against greed (Luke 12:15).
- To those whom much is given will much be expected (Luke 12:48)
- There are serious consequences for those who swindle people who seek God (Matthew 21:12).
- True treasure is found in serving others rather than being wealthy (Luke 18:22).
- Genuine giving involves sacrifice (Mark 12:42–44).

Successful aging involves wise stewardship for personal, inter-personal, and environmental balance, as well as intellectual, emotional, and spiritual health. We are stewards: caretakers given responsibility for ourselves, our relationships, our world, and all that is around us. Both the journey and the venue are a part of the process in which we explore and discover what it is to live as wise stewards and whole people of God. Genesis proclaims that we are not meant to be alone—a declaration of our inter-connectedness and human need for relationship, not a mandate for marriage as some have interpreted it to be.[22] A part of wholeness, well-being, and successful aging is cultivating relationships with others and with God. For Christians, the living example and redemptive relationship of Jesus with humanity embodies the essence of what we need to know about stewardship of life and wholeness of living.

Jesus celebrated children, healed the infirm, honored the aged, rejoiced at a party, fed the hungry, confronted obstacles, prayed with fervor, sought renewal in isolation, chose the neglected, acknowledged his humanity, challenged his intellect, and laughed at the absurd. For those who find it surprising that I mention Jesus laughing at the absurd, I find it hard to imagine someone with no sense of humor creating metaphors about camels passing through the eye of a needle; however one might interpret that passage![23] He demonstrated life as something to be embraced, celebrated, and cherished while also pointing to the eternal and transcendent. Stewardship of life is a crucial part of our perspective of well-being and successful aging.

If we see each day as a blessing and opportunity, we will likely do a better job of cherishing that day and living in the present. An octogenarian I knew always greeted each new day with excitement and a smile. He said that when he took life for what it was as it came along, rather than having mountaintop expectations for every day, he was rarely disappointed. At first, I thought this to be a rather negative perspective, but I came to understand what he meant. He chose to live in the present moment. He saw life as a gift and his role as a steward of that gift. He waited for each day to unfold as it would, instead of expecting that everyday must be wonderful and full of only fun and excitement. He knew that, good or bad, each day held both opportunity and possibility. He trusted that whatever the day might bring, God would be at work, even in the trying times, to give him something great each day. As a result, he lived life with a genuine sense of gratitude for blessings and challenges. He discovered lessons to be learned from days of difficulty. His gratitude for life overflowed in a wise and generous stewardship of life, such that he made a financial fortune through diligence, thrift, and generosity.

It is said that a closed fist cannot receive. The Dead Sea is one of the lowest spots on the planet, excluding the ocean depths, at 1,300 feet below sea level. It is dead because the waters of the Jordan River flow into it, but nothing flows out of it. Minerals and salts accumulate in the sea and make it almost uninhabitable. When we open our lives to allow possibilities to flow in and blessings to flow out, we embrace life as an opportunity for blessing, service, and joy. We discover that to be whole and live well is to be aware of and connected to our bodies, our minds, our spirit, our world, our relationships, our dreams, our hopes, and our God.

Stewardship of life grasps the reality that life is a gift and that we do not possess things but are entrusted with them. The lives of people around us are also a sacred trust. When we strive for peace by listening to others, acknowledging their needs, and understanding their desires, we bring about wholeness of life which is the path of peace. Peace is achievable and poverty can be eliminated when we envision a world that strives to make it so and then act to do our part. A sense of stewardship is a sense of responsibility to be caregivers and caretakers as wise sages have taught, and Jesus has exemplified.

Choose to Focus on Others' Needs

America is a nation built by devotion, perseverance, and service, but according to the Bureau of Labor Statistics, the overall number of Americans who offer voluntary service is declining. Roughly one in four Americans who volunteer give more than an hour per week for a worthy cause, with those who are older than sixty-four giving twice that amount. From 2003 to 2005, the percentage of volunteers among the total population remained constant at 28.8%, but by 2007 that number slipped to 26.2%. When you translate the percentages into people (approximately 800,000 fewer volunteers) and the decrease in volunteer hours (at least one million fewer volunteer hours) the loss takes on almost staggering proportions.[24] Though some of the diminished number of volunteers can be explained by the increase in dual-income households and people working past the typical age of retirement, the rise of retiring Baby Boomers (who actually retire or reduce working hours) should ease such decline, but it has not.

Focusing on the needs of others rather than dwelling on our own circumstances is an essential coping skill of healthy aging that has a positive influence on mind, body, and spirit. The sense of satisfaction and fulfillment that comes from selfless service helps to reduce stress, strengthen the immune system, and enhance our sense of well-being. Service to others brings a sense of fulfillment from seeing our lives in a greater and purposeful context while allowing us to draw satisfaction from completing objectives, providing a service, and addressing the needs of people and organizations around us.

A serious discussion on the benefit of looking beyond ourselves and growing beyond our human tendency to be merely self-focused and self-centered, must also address our fear of putting the needs of others above our own. Never growing beyond self-centeredness is rooted in human selfishness and spiritual laziness. In adults, it is a sign of immaturity of thought and spirit. It usually begins with the fear of not having enough or not having all that we want. One common fear of people whom I interviewed was the fear of outliving their financial resources. It is certain that we are living longer and many people who made their financial plans decades ago did not anticipate how many years their retirement savings would need to span. The National Center for Health Statistics in Atlanta, Georgia, a part of the Centers for Disease Control and Prevention, states in a 2009 report that life expectancy in the United States now averages nearly seventy-eight years— an all-time high since such data was compiled.[25]

Financially, most could not anticipate the severe economic recession and devastating monetary losses brought on by unbridled corporate greed, blatant financial fraud, and the collapse of the home mortgage market. With increased cost of living, skyrocketing fuel costs, and decreased interest rates, financial fears can be genuine and understandable. It would be idealistic to say that money doesn't matter, just as it is for a newlywed couple to say, "We can live on love alone." As the old adage goes in reply to that naïve affirmation, "Love don't [sic] taste like bread!"

Still, there is something confining and myopic about narrowing our focus to money and possessions as we grow older. Some of it comes from the expectation of an inheritance on the part of our children and grandchildren. We may want to please others, or desire others to like or admire us. Money and possessions can influence others, but it yields a shallow affirmation that does not reflect true appreciation.

Possessions can also evoke a false sense of security. The importance we place on material things is truly our choosing, and tangible goods may bring certain feelings of assurance or comfort, but those feelings are our own. An old, orange life-preserver may get tossed on the fifty-cent pile at a garage sale, but it is priceless if you are aboard the Titanic as she begins to sink! One thing is clear, no matter how we philosophically talk about materialism and possessions: we like our "stuff." We want to be surrounded by our "stuff." When we run out of room where we live, rather than divest ourselves of our "stuff," we pay to store it elsewhere. We pay to protect it by alarming our residence, our garage, our warehouse and our cars. We pay to insure it, and when we lose it through fire, theft, or other calamity, we will pay again (the insurance company calls it a "deductible") in order to get it back and then some. How much simpler life is when we relinquish all of that!

Money is great to have and power feels good, but the most powerful people I have ever met were not extrinsically wealthy but were powerful of spirit. I have encountered towering intellects who convincingly declared that there is no God and that life is all happenstance. What I often saw behind their intelligence and sophistry was an emptiness and isolation. I have sat in the twelfth-floor office of a CEO who made just under a million dollar salary in a "bad year" and heard ego and bravado, but little true power. He went to the "right church," belonged to the "right organizations," and donated just enough to get a charitable deduction on his taxes. He was financially secure and spiritually bankrupt.

Repeatedly, those who place their focus on others and service beyond self have a sense of stewardship and maturity that yields a healthy spirit and an inner strength that adds to longevity and well-being. There is wellness in living as whole people, and wholeness can be found when concern for others is lifted above self-centeredness while humbly acknowledging our own needs. We really do receive by giving ourselves away. A closed fist cannot receive.

Focusing on the needs of others yields a life of love, service, optimism, generosity, and joy. Think about the sort of person with whom you enjoy spending time. Optimistic, joyful, loving people are more alive than those concerned with how they look and what sort of impression they make. Wise, outward-focused people see life as adventure, art, opportunity, and celebration. Relationships are new occasions for personal development, life enhancement, intellectual renewal, stereotype shattering, self-awareness, human discovery, and horizon expansion. Life is a bank and God has given us the key to the vault. So why spend our time holding on to our own lock-box when we can see what else there is to explore?

Perhaps one other-focused relationship that many people have is far more beneficial than we might realize. If you are a pet owner, having that special relationship can add to your longevity. Vanessa Gisquet, of *Forbes.com* reports:

> According to *Public Health Reports*, a study done in 1980 showed that the survival rates of heart attack victims who

had a pet were twenty-eight percent higher than those of patients who didn't have an animal companion. "The health effects seem to be very real and by no means mystical," says Alan Beck, director of the Center for the Human-Animal Bond at Purdue University. "Contact with companion animals triggers a relaxation response," he says.

Rebecca Johnson, a professor of gerontological nursing at the University of Missouri at Columbia, showed that interaction with pets does, in fact, reduce levels of the stress hormone cortisol. The ability of companion pets to reduce our overall stress level probably accounts for most of their life-extending qualities. "For many people, pets also provide a reason to get moving," adds Johnson. How many people, after all, would actually get any exercise if it weren't for their over-enthusiastic dog?[26]

Consider your life, your attitude, and your relationships. Do you tend to be more self-centered or selfless? Do you tend to be focused inwardly or on the world and people around you? Inquire of others who know you well and ask how they perceive you. Explore these questions/scenarios, reflecting on them individually or as a group:

- If you lived in an apartment complex and your unit caught fire, would you first save a possession before warning your neighbors?

- If you had adequate time to save one possession in your home from some pending disaster, what would you save?

- Is the possession you would save something that has sentimental value (relationship-oriented) or monetary value (financially-oriented)?

- If you listed ten things that you value most in life, how many are relationships, accomplishments, things, memories or something about yourself (e.g. health)?

I especially like this quote from Reverend Douglas Fitch, Senior Pastor of Glide Memorial United Methodist Church in San Francisco. Glide is a vibrant and amazing inner-city church that ministers to the wayward homeless and the well-off celebrity. From ministry to AIDS patients to counting movie stars among its congregation, the church is a transforming presence in that city. Speaking at a conference on ministry to adults and the aged, Fitch said, "Conviction is worthless unless it is converted into conduct."[27] Life is not only about what we believe, but how we act upon those beliefs. Actions and words give integrity to each other.

For Reflection

1. Do you identify with one or more of the three Principles?

2. Do you think that anxiety about aging is worse for "Baby Boomers" and subsequent generations than it was for those born prior to 1943 who endured World Wars and the Great Depression?

3. Considering only American culture, do you feel that Americans are becoming less narcissistic and more caring of others than we once were? Considering humanity as a whole, do you think that there is more or less anxiety today than during the era termed, "The Cold War?" How does this relate to fear of growing older?

A FRESH
PERSPECTIVE

Stepping Back for a Different View

"I really liked the new guy I met online, until I actually met him."

—Anonymous E-dater

"Don't confuse being 'soft' with seeing the other guys point of view."

—George H. W. Bush,
"All the Best, George Bush"

"Perpetual optimism is a force multiplier."

—Former Secretary of State Colin Powell
U.S. Army General (Retired)
and former Chairman of the Joint Chiefs

Examining Our Perspective

We have looked at the first of the "Three P's" of successful aging: Principles, the values to which we anchor ourselves. Before we can formulate our plan for aging well, we move from our Principles to examine our Perspective. To maintain a healthy and balanced Perspective, it is essential that we:

- Keep an attitude of optimism
- Enjoy a sense of humor
- Nurture a spiritual perspective

Keep an Attitude of Optimism

If you are an optimist, you will be happy to learn that you will likely live longer. In 2002, researchers at the Mayo Clinic in Rochester, Minnesota, found that optimistic people decreased their risk of early death by fifty percent, compared with those who leaned more toward pessimism. Reporting on this study, writer Vanessa Gisquet commented, "If you really want to live longer, then you can start with your attitude. Your way of thinking can not only impact the quality of your life, but also how long you actually live."[28]

"The exact mechanism of how personality acts as a risk factor for early death or poorer health is unclear," says Dr. Toshihiko Maruta, the main investigator in the study. Most likely, it has to do with the fact that pessimists have an increased chance for future problems with their physical health, career achievements, and emotional stress—particularly depression. "Yet another possibility could be more directly biological, like changes in the immune system," Maruta adds.[29]

Bob Arnot, M.D., popular physician of radio and television fame as well as a columnist for *Men's Journal*, suggests two sources every pessimist must read. He writes:

> If you're trying to turn the corner, start by reading Seligman's *Learned Optimism* or my book, *The Biology of Success*, which teach how to change belief systems in ways that allow for more constructive personal habits ... Martin Seligman is an American psychologist who has been studying the effects of pessimism for more than a quarter of a century. He believes pessimism is a learned trait that is intrinsically related to depression. On the upside, both can be thwarted by changing your beliefs and learning how to gain power over negative situations.[30]

One of the greatest barriers to living life to our fullest potential is our tendency to be afraid, pessimistic, or self-defeating. People tend to bring about that which they believe will come true. If you think that your life cannot get any better, your prediction will likely become self-fulfilling; you have thought your way into the reality you experience. If you think that your actions and attitude can have a positive impact on your life, your future and your world, then you will likely work to make it so, and they will.

Live with true optimism and reconsider your life by taking a step back so that you can gain a fresh and positive perspective. Aging need not be a reason for pessimism and gloom. God is looking at the future and smiling, for God knows that there is both joy and blessing ahead. Optimism gives birth to hope and a hopeful heart sustains an optimistic spirit. It is one of the healthiest examples of symbiosis you may ever find!

You may be in a difficult place now. There may not be anything positive yet visible on the horizon. Hope may seem naïve or simplistic, but true hope is neither. Hope is grounded in the fundamental faith in a God whose grace and redemption are more powerful than evil and destruction. Keep living large and thinking great things, because optimism is to life what water is to parched ground, a nourishing source of transformation.

Your life will unfold as it will. Aging is a part of that unfolding, and it will also bring benefits which are not yet foreseen. You can grow older without fear when you live with optimism that is rooted in faith. God is already at work for good in the lives of all who would claim God's power, hope, and peace.

Keep this thought in mind:

Optimism looks with promise toward an unseen future while celebrating the blessing of the present.

If you are facing a debilitating illness, handicap, divorce, or other difficult time, it is important to understand what this sentence can mean to you. The gift of this day—this present moment—as difficult a time as it may be, has yet to be appreciated, fulfilled, or understood without the perspective of tomorrow. Have faith that God is at work in spite of the difficulties of today, just as certainly as God is looking at the future and smiling with the surety of the hope that lies ahead. God knows what is to come, and knows that there are better days and greater blessings still to be realized.

An attitude of optimism about life and growing older breeds hope and possibility. Hope is a powerful force and a conscious choice. The poet, Emily Dickinson, who battled mental illness and depression, was still able to write these words of hope:

Hope is a strange invention—
A Patent of the Heart—
In unremitting action
Yet never wearing out.[31]

On another occasion, she penned these words:

> Hope is a thing with feathers
> That perches in the soul
> And sings a tune without the words
> And never stops at all...[32]

Hope looks at life from a larger perspective and dwells content in the knowledge that God can bring something redemptive out of even the grayest of days. Optimism is not naïve, every-thing-is-always-going-to-be-okay thinking. True optimism is rooted in faith and hope that looks to the future and sees possibility and promise.

You and I know of many people who have every reason not to be optimistic, yet they have an outlook that pierces through looming darkness like a halogen spotlight. I still have a greeting card that was sent to me a few months after my youngest son, John, was born. Many cards and letters of good wishes were received, but this one was so significant that I pull it out occasionally just to read it again. It was from Berniece, a senior adult who I had gotten to know at the time of her husband's illness and death when I lived in a small community outside of Fort Worth. The card informed me that Berniece was involved in a terrible car accident about the time of John's birth that had left her badly injured. She spent weeks in the hospital, still more weeks in a specialty hospital, several more in a rehabilitation hospital, and then some recovery time in an assisted living center before being able to return to her home. During the more critical days following her accident, her son died. She was unable to be aware of his death, and so was not informed until many days after the service that had been held in his memory.

She had every reason to be bitter, angry, or withdrawn, and certainly there were dark and difficult days. During her recovery, when she was still unable to get around without assistance, Berniece asked a friend to purchase a greeting card to celebrate the birth of our son. Her friend purchased, addressed, and added the proper postage, but Berniece insisted upon personally writing a message with the card, despite a painfully broken wrist that was splinted.

She shared what had happened, apologized if her story sounded as if she was complaining, thanked God for new life in the form of John's birth, and simply asked for prayers as she continued to heal. It was not a brief note, as her writing filled the lower half of the card below the printed greeting, spilled over to the inside flap, and then continued on the back of the card. In her injury-induced shaky penmanship, she conveyed the reality of her condition and the optimism of her spirit. My eyes welled with tears as I returned the card to its envelope, only then noticing the return address. Berniece resided on Hope Drive!

Optimism can give birth to hope and a hopeful heart sustains an optimistic spirit. It does not always seem logical, the circumstances of hope may seem anachronistic and the grounding of hope may indeed be miraculous. Such is the nature of a miracle. A miracle points to the holy: the presence of God. Hope sings a tune when there are no words and casts the positive light of optimism where only pessimism and despair are thought to dwell.

Keep an attitude of optimism and you will find your life surrounded by positive people, filled with much success, and overflowing with abundant hope.

Enjoy a Sense of Humor

Humor is a vital component to healthy aging. Having a sense of humor is not the same as being optimistic, though most optimists tend to also have an ability to laugh at the tribulations and trials of life. The noted comedian, Robin Williams, distinguished humor from optimism when he said, "Comedy is acting out optimism."[33]

Humor embraces the absurd and the hilarious. It births laughter that catches the oppressor off-guard, robs trouble of its despondency, and lightens the burdens of the beleaguered. Good humor helps us to take ourselves less seriously and casts a brighter light on the darker days of woe. Humor celebrates the joy of life.

Humor, too, is a gift of God to the human experience. It can be born of the absurd occurrence, surprising spontaneity, the comic juxtaposition of current events and situations, or the wry wit of a keen intellect. It can come from the ability to see irony in a variety of circumstances or from the precious gift of not taking one's self too seriously. One of the reasons that slapstick comedy endures is its self-deprecating humor. When humor is selfless rather than mean-spirited or sarcastic, it is much more delightful. When we cultivate the ability to laugh at ourselves and find humor amidst life's challenges and difficulties, our journey of living will be much lighter and far more enjoyable.

Late night talk shows, such as NBC's *The Tonight Show* and CBS's *The Late Show with David Letterman*, use humor and fun as the vehicle of their entertainment focus. They have been so successful because so many people look to humor to close out their day. After the challenges and failures of a long day, the delight of humor is the salve that comforts. Humor that pokes fun at the world's woes, the politically powerful, the celebrated movie star, our own lives, or even at the comedians themselves, puts life in perspective and gives us the ability to laugh at ourselves. When a joke "bombs," even the failure can become humorous and helps to put a different angle on our own failures. Laughter is therapeutic. Norman Cousin's classic book, *Anatomy of an Illness as Perceived by the Patient*, demonstrates this great truth.[34]

Cousins was quite ill with a poor prognosis. He arranged to have taped programs of comedians such as The Three Stooges, Charlie Chaplin, and Red Skelton brought to his room, and he watched them daily. The laughter that these great comedians triggered welled-up in his soul and strengthened his spirit and his body. He began to feel better. For him, laughter was truly the medicine that he required. Given Cousin's experience, it is not surprising that when I served as a hospital chaplain, I observed how patients with a sense of humor and a spirit of optimism fared better and often recovered more swiftly than those who dwelt on their own pain and woes.

According to an article from the Society for Neuroscience, ongoing research lends even more scientific credence to this observation:

> Currently, researchers are trying to further understand the precise roles that different brain areas play and how their functions may overlap. They also want to determine how the processing [of humor] may tie to disease. For example, scientists plan to examine the activity of depressed people to see if their humor processing ability is impaired. If it is, then boosting the system's activity may help depression.
>
> Already some small studies hint that the brain activity from humor may have a medical benefit. For example, human tests have found some evidence that humorous videos and tapes can reduce feelings of pain, prevent nega-

tive stress reactions and boost the brain's biological battle against infection."[35]

Initial studies reveal that humor involves three separate areas of brain activity. Cognitive processing comprehends the joke, motor processing triggers the muscles involved in smiling and laughter, and emotional processing generates the good feelings of happiness and fun.[36]

Brain research has also revealed that humor has a genuine effect on brain plasticity, the ability for the brain to reorganize and create new neuropathways throughout its lifespan. Humor is conceptual, triggering associations that evoke a response. This explains why something may be raucously funny for some individuals and not humorous for others. Perspective, experience, associations, personality, and individual taste are all factors that determine whether a particular joke or comic routine is funny to an audience. Ask any comedian who tries to "work a dead room." If the audience is not laughing, the comedian has not connected to the mental associations and factors peculiar to that particular crowd, without which it is hard to build momentum and achieve comedic success.

My own experience, and perhaps yours as well, makes personal what clinical behavioral study documents: people of good humor help make life delightful. One of the best examples from my youth is also a cherished memory that I carry with me to this day. Her name was Elizabeth Williams, and she masterfully taught English Literature at my high school until her retirement my senior year. I wish to add, in my defense, that her retirement was planned and had nothing to do with having me as a student, though she would playfully dispute that argument!

Ms. Williams was either a notorious or a popular high school

English teacher, depending upon your perspective. She was a no-nonsense, West Texas ranching woman who commuted to Fort Worth from the rural cattle and oil community of Jacksboro, Texas. I still can hear her deep and booming baritone voice that could stop you in your tracks, and her often infectious laugh that caught you by surprise then gave you a reason to join in. After I had asked one-too-many questions about a class assignment, she looked at me and began to quote Shakespeare, "Out damn'd spot!" I didn't get it at the time, but later—much, much later—looked back on that day with the same laughter that was aimed at me by my classmates at the time.

She waxed poetic in her more reflective moods, speaking of retirement, aging, and the next phase of her journey. As the year was winding down and her last week of classroom teaching arrived, she seemed to soften and get misty-eyed. She was more generous with her hugs, discounting the affection they conveyed by saying, "You can hug everyone when you're old because people think that you are just starved for sex!"

Mrs. Williams taught me that laughter can come from surprising people at surprising times. It can be the delightful giggle of a playful child, the raucous laughter of a boisterous youth, or a poet-loving English teacher with a sense of humor that I did not grasp until it was almost too late. The humor of life is where one finds it, and is a gift of the human experience that lifts the spirit, lightens the burden, and sometimes heals what nothing else can.

The phrase, "to enjoy a sense of humor," carries its own feeling of pleasure and delight. Humor is the stuff of which life's "fun" is made. It is one of life's best ingredients. You don't stop laughing because you grow old; you grow old because you stop laughing.

Nurture a Spiritual Perspective

Healthy aging takes a holistic view of the human condition and understands that body and spirit are interrelated. We already know that the systems within our physical body are related. For example, if we wish to not neglect our heart, we need also not neglect our teeth. My dentist, Dr. Kent Mach, once explained to me how inadequate dental hygiene can lead to complications possibly resulting in an infection that, if left untreated, can impair the heart and other organs. I tried to use this logic to convince my youngest son to brush his teeth without being prompted, but I wasn't successful. Still, just as our heart and our mouth are more closely connected than we might realize or accept, there is a connection between body and spirit.

A spiritual perspective looks at life from a transcendent point of view and puts in broader context the troubles of the moment with the larger picture of the journey. A spiritual perspective places faith and trust in that which is unseen and has a greater capacity to overcome setbacks and heartache. A spiritual perspective holds fast to hope and brings both peace and blessing to the journey of life.

Body and soul are both components vital to healthy living whose mutual development and care should not be ignored. One of the basic steps of any twelve-step program of addiction recovery is to acknowledge our dependence upon a higher power, however one defines that power. My life experience tells me that God is real, and God's power and grace—God's unconditional love—are gifts we have only to claim in order to receive. God is never pushy, so we must be the one to open the door, seek the Truth, search for the Way, believe, and celebrate. God comes knocking, but only we can choose to open the door of our heart and life to let God's presence abide there. There is an emptiness in life that only a Divine relationship can fulfill.

Making such a connection between the corporeal and the spiritual is more difficult for some. As a pastoral counselor integrating spirituality and psychotherapy, I have had clients who were in a twelve-step recovery program who found the spiritual dimension of the program a difficult concept to grasp. Some clients viewed the reality of life as only that which could be empirically measured and experienced, and so the abstract and ethereal realm of spirituality, which requires faith, was elusive. For others, their only experience of a Higher Power was abusive religion or news accounts of terrorists whose sadistically twisted religious fervor resulted in the death and maiming of thousands of innocents. Some grew up in cruelty, spawned by a horribly destructive religious belief system adopted by their parents and/or grandparents. Some had been abused by religious leaders in whom they had been taught to place their complete trust and obedience. To help such wounded people discern bad religion from healthy spirituality is a formidable, but vitally worthwhile task. Faith in God cannot be measured, but the experience of such faith is immeasurable in value.

In a ten-year, $2.4 million study, primarily funded by the John Templeton Foundation, 1,800 patients who underwent heart bypass surgery were studied for a relationship between prayer and healing. One-third of the patients were prayed for without their knowledge, while one-third were prayed for with their knowledge. The other third of the patients were not included in the prayers of the faith groups involved. In this study, those who were prayed for with their knowledge and consent experienced slightly higher complications than did the other two groups. Is prayer not efficacious at all, or as

Dr. Charles Bethea, a cardiologist and co-author of the study observed, "Did the patients think, 'I am so sick that they had to call in the prayer team?'"

For the faith groups involved, the study was either disappointing or, as Dr. David Stevens, Executive Director of the Christian Medical and Dental Association said, "the scientists were not equipped to measure the phenomenon." As theologians have pointed out, to directly correlate healing with each individual prayer implies that we control God to assure a specific outcome.[37]

Though this study may dismay some in the spiritual community while being used as fodder for atheistic viewpoints, it does not speak a final word on the power of having a spiritual perspective. Pierre Teilhard de Chardin, a French theologian and paleontologist (1881–1955), said, "We are not human beings having a spiritual experience, but we are spiritual beings having a human experience."[38] We are spiritual beings on a physical journey and a transcendent viewpoint yields greater understanding and a sense of peace.

I do not know of a major U.S. hospital that does not have a chaplain, whether on staff or a volunteer, to tend to the spiritual needs of patients. A chaplain listens, prays, and offers a transcendent perception that yields hope when an immanent view sees only despair. It is not a childish hope or a hope of denial, but rather a hope of possibility that sees the present as only a small part of a greater tapestry that is beautiful, redemptive, and purposeful.

In the early days of tribal medicine, spiritual men and women were often considered healers within the tribe. Spirituality and the healing of the body were interwoven. In spite of the limitations of ancient medicine, there were also many successes through the wisdom of herbal medicine and spiritual blessing that brought healing and peace, and allowed the body's own immune system to work by lessening anxiety. Medical science continues to explore the vital interrelationship between body and spirit, but to measure what may be immeasurable complicates such understanding.

Body and spirit are interrelated; this awareness makes a vital contribution to healthy aging. Spiritually strong people are not guaranteed a life without health struggles, but they will be better equipped to address whatever obstacles they may face because of their spiritual perspective. It is also worth noting that some of the greatest minds and souls of history have used the power of their spirit and intellect to transcend the limitations of their body. Ludwig von Beethoven, who was profoundly deaf, believed that in heaven he would at last be able to hear his musical works. Helen Keller, left both blind and deaf following an illness in her infancy, gave thanks to God for the miracle of her amazing life's journey.

You may choose not to believe in a spiritual aspect to life. You may desire empirical evidence to prove that it even exists. Your concept of spirituality may be very different than others and you may not believe in God or any Higher Power at all. We are an amazingly diverse people in a wondrously diverse universe. Our tremendous diversity gives depth and breadth to the divinely created gift of life, while our humanity keeps us all connected. Lack of belief in a Higher Power does not change the truth of that reality any more than lack of belief in gravity will make you fly. True and redemptive spirituality cannot be boiled down to simply a set of rules or a quantitative and qualifying checklist. This may be disturbing to some, but it need not be. God knows that rules cannot ultimately satisfy, nor can qualifications alone measure our faith.

True, fulfilling and redemptive spirituality that is our compass for living has but one requirement: a relationship with God. Only a relationship with God can satisfy our search for ultimate fulfillment and lead us to the answer of the question we all ask, "Why am I here?" We want to solve the mystery of finding our purpose. A relationship with the Divine allows us to realize that it is in the love and acceptance of others and ourselves that we find our true fulfillment and purpose. Spirituality is always rooted in faith that goes beyond what we can prove or measure. God, our creator, redeemer, and compass, points us toward a way of living that we might offer the gracious love, compassionate kindness, and unconditional acceptance to others that we have been given, while humbly serving as we have humbly received.

Spirituality is about transcendent love and relationship, not condemnation and judgment. In our rush to condemn, we humans have created enough pain and sorrow to fill a thousand hells. Some have insisted that others adhere to their interpretation of Holy Scripture and by their action have made life miserable for those not accepting the same interpretation. Slavery was supported from the pulpit and the pew by Christians misapplying and abusing the scriptures. Some white supremacists use the same tactics today. Countless women through the centuries have been subjugated, rejected, tortured, or put to death as a result of patriarchal or even misogynistic interpretations that have denied them the leadership roles to which they have been called. There are still those who refuse to let women teach or preach to men in churches and seminaries, singling them out solely because of their gender, regardless of their gifts. Gay, lesbian, or transgender individuals have been the brunt of religious anger or even violence spawned by an out-of-context or superficial reading of ancient scripture. The Apostle Paul's condemnation of homosexual pederasty or debauchery among Greeks and Romans has no correlation to a loving, monogamous, and committed gay couple simply seeking to live their life in peace.

One significant problem of a rigid, dogmatic approach to scripture is to discern where emphasis should be placed and our energies focused. Since adultery is such a significant and genuine threat to marriage, why is it not the focus of major public debate, legislation, and doctrinal enforcement and given the same energy and attention that is directed to homosexuality? If we are to take seriously the great commission to go and make disciples of all nations (Matthew 28:18–20), then why not ordain women to the priesthood since there is such a global shortage of priests and so many women waiting to serve? Those who focus on rigid dogma and condemnation and define God in such terms are missing the theology of grace: God's unconditional love. Redemption and grace are the mark of divine love, which leads me to one final word about nurturing a spiritual perspective: Forgiveness!

Relationships are messy. We can have good intentions and still be hurtful, whether out of carelessness, callousness, or ignorance. Sometimes we are simply mean-spirited, self-centered, or more interested in being "right" (winning) than being happy (contented). Some of us enjoy winning at the expense of another, and I am not speaking of competitive sports or academics. Sometimes we inflict harm and ignore the consequences.

Forgiveness is a component of the transcendent. It is more than a mere emotional release, although anger can be assuaged. Forgiveness is more than an intellectual exercise, although it involves conscious choice. Forgiveness rises above human pettiness and the tawdry behavior of exploitation, greed, and control, or the despicable behavior of violence, negligence, and injustice. In the last half of my ministry as a parish pastor, I realized that there is one point in life's journey where forgiveness is especially crucial: whenever we face death and our own mortality. As a result, I spoke about forgiveness at every funeral or memorial service and received words of gratitude from those in attendance every time I did so.

In every family and in almost every human relationship, there are things that we regret having said or that we failed to say, or actions we regret having done or failed to do. At a time of death and farewell to a loved one or friend, it is important that we allow these regrets to be released and to die as well. When the funeral cortege reaches its end for the final committal service at the cemetery, I have often said these eight simple words to all those gathered around the open grave: "Remember what it is that we bury today."

It is only a body that we bury. "Ashes to ashes and dust to dust," as the Book of Common Prayer so beautifully phrases the meaning of Genesis 3:19 and Ecclesiastes 3:20.[39] We bury what is finite and commend the spirit of our loved one to infinite realm of God's love and care. We take with us the precious memories, sacred moments, and joyous laughter that is always ours to hold close and that death can never grasp. There are other things that we need to bury: that which we said or did that we wished we could "undo," and that which we failed to say or do before the time had gone. These need also be laid to rest, buried, and never dug up again.

Forgiving ourselves and forgiving each other is essential for healthy living and successful aging. We do well when we approach life as Norman Cousins declares: "Life is an adventure in forgiveness."[40] We discover transcendent opportunities to grow in spirit and in our knowledge of unconditional love, so that along with growing older, we might grow wiser as well.

For Reflection

1. Do you consider yourself an optimistic person? Do optimism and humor play a role in helping you face difficulties in your life? Although humor is healthy, consider if you or someone you know may use humor to mask or ignore, rather than transcend, difficulties or challenges. Consider such signs as laughing inappropriately or excessively, or frequent use of self-deprecating humor.

2. Norman Vincent Peale once said, "Change your thoughts and you change your world." What unhelpful thoughts or attitudes do you need to change in order to develop a healthier perspective on life?

3. The Twelve Steps of Alcoholics Anonymous emphasizes the acknowledgment of a Higher Power "as we understand him [her]." Reflect upon your belief (or disbelief) in God or a Higher Power. How does faith and spirituality play a role in your life, your outlook, and your relationships?

MAKING A PLAN

Self-Care, Your Network, and Your Vision

"It takes a long time to grow young."

—Pablo Picasso

"As for me, I have no sense of chronology, or age. I must have a screw loose, because I live my life day to day."

—Ben Kingsley[41]

"He who every morning plans the transaction of the day and follows out that plan, carries a thread that will guide him through the maze of the most busy life. But where no plan is laid, where the disposal of time is surrendered merely to the chance of incidence, chaos will soon reign."

—Victor Hugo

Your Plan

After *Principles* and *Perspective* comes the concrete making of a *Plan*. A Plan for successful aging includes committing to specific actions for self-care, developing a supportive network, and formulating a clear vision for the future toward which we wish to move and live. Succinctly, the third "P" of aging well urges us to:

- Make a Plan of Self-Care
- Develop a Supportive Network
- Hold a Vision for the Future

Make a Plan of Self-Care

People who set goals for themselves accomplish more. They are men and women on a mission. Australian gold-medalist swimmer, Ian Thorpe, was quoted by print media saying that American swimming great, Michael Phelps, would never be able to beat Mark Spitz's seven-gold medal performance in the 1972 Munich Olympic games. Phelps taped the article to the back of his locker for motivation. It became his goal to do just that, and the result was the incredible eight gold medals the swimming phenomenon collected at the 2008 Beijing games.[42] People who set goals accomplish more than those who do not. This also applies to self-care and successful aging.

Though putting something in writing with clearly defined and measurable goals is ideal, a plan of self-care may not be a formally written plan or even a spoken one. Though most of us need the discipline of writing out a plan in a concrete way, what an effective plan *must* be is intentional. An intentional plan means a conscious acknowledgment of and commitment to the need and desire to become healthy and to adopt a healthy lifestyle. Self-care includes at least annual medical exams by a physician or other health-care practitioner, with particular health screenings based on age and gender (see Tables 1–3). A family history of certain diseases, such as diabetes or breast cancer, may require earlier and more frequent exams. Nutrition, exercise, education, spirituality, motivation, self-awareness, and fun are all crucial to a plan of self-care. What is the use of having a plan to live longer if you don't have fun along the way?

Enjoyment, significance, relationship, and self-improvement are all necessary for our life to be meaningful, fun, exciting, and productive. These are what move us from surviving to thriving. It reminds me of the joke about the fifty-something-year-old man who was hit by a car and awoke to discover that he had died and was in heaven. He said aloud when he realized his situation, "If I had known I was only going to live this long, I would have eaten less bran and enjoyed more cheesecake." Self-care involves self-discipline, which brings to mind the oft-repeated Nike slogan, "No pain, no gain;" in other words, self-discipline costs you something. Self-care is also motivated by results that make our efforts worthwhile and enjoyment that brings fun and satisfaction along the way.

Climbing on a treadmill became drudgery for me. I varied the routine a bit, joined a fitness club, and took advantage of their elliptical trainers, stair-climbing machines, stationary bicycles, rowing and weight-training equipment. I bought some headphones to listen to music or to CNN and the morning shows on large screen TV's. When that became tedious, I got a bicycle from a pawn shop and enjoyed riding in my neighborhood. I walked community trails with friends, went swimming, jogging, or just enjoyed a walk in my neighborhood. I was feeling guilty for not being better-disciplined, so I took advantage of a personal trainer for a month. The trainer not only pushed me to better and consistent fitness performance, he taught me what I needed to know and continue to do after my sessions with him were completed so that I could maintain my results. I soon was in the best shape of my life and I was in my late forties. Of course, I couldn't afford to keep a personal trainer, and motivation eventually waned as my schedule fluctuated. Trying to stay healthy and fit just wasn't as much fun anymore.

Finally, I realized that I didn't have to do one thing all of the time in order to be healthy, it was only important that I do *something* that gave my heart a workout, energized me with my own body's natural endorphins, strengthened my muscles and bones, and moved my joints to keep my body in motion for ongoing health. Drudgery became welcomed opportunity when I wasn't exercising because I needed to, but because I wanted to. I felt better, slept better, and was happier.

No matter our plan or efforts toward health, there are components impacting health and longevity that are beyond our control or self-discipline, with genetics being the most obvious obstacle—for now. Though genetic research will ultimately make it possible to manipulate and eradicate certain birth defects or genetic dispositions such as Down Syndrome or Multiple Sclerosis, we are constrained by our genes and family history. Because of this truth, I don't use the phrase "staying healthy," but rather becoming healthy; that is, moving toward healthy habits and choices. It is an ongoing process and a life-long lifestyle for wellness and successful aging.

There may be other factors that limit our healthy choices and behavior, such as our environment, economics, geography, and culture. Those living in economic poverty may have a more difficult time maintaining their health because of a lack of affordable healthcare, nutrition, transportation, proper clothing, or energy for heating or cooling their homes. In metropolitan Dallas, Texas, a city of billionaires, vast community resources, and numerous social services for the poor, disabled, and aged, there are still people who die each year from excessive heat or cold because they cannot afford the energy to cool or heat their homes. Similarly, those living in remote areas may not have ready access to basic healthcare, medical knowledge, nutritional information, mental health resources, and staple groceries that many of us take for granted in our pantry. Poverty is real and forever leaves its mark, even upon those who are able to overcome it.

Self-care is about improving and maintaining quality of life. Health is encompassing of body, mind, and spirit. Aging is not limited to physical changes, but also to changing emotional, intellectual, and spiritual needs. Significant personal growth can come through all manner of self-care. Improving one's self by resolving inner conflict through counseling, seeking career change or higher education, exploring and deepening one's spirituality, making time in your life for hobbies or special interests, cultivating relationships with others, belonging to a service organization, attending a singles or couples group, or taking advantage of marriage/relationship enrichment opportunities are all means of self-care.

Renewal comes in many forms. Remind yourself that the word "recreation" means to be *re-created* or made new or whole once more. Celebrate times of renewal, and journey often down whatever path leads to that place for you that is a means of self-care.

What stops you from taking better care of yourself? If a lack of self-discipline is your "Achilles' heel," then consider these ways of motivating you toward your goals.

- Have a plan. The more intentional you are about your health, the more likely it is that you will take some action and the greater quality of life you will have.

- Set specific, realistic, and measurable goals (e.g. I will lose ten pounds in two months; I will spend ten minutes each day in quiet reflection; I will join and attend a yoga class for five weeks).

- Get a workout partner, walking companion, or join an exercise class.

- If you are unable to find an exercise or walking group, organize one by inviting neighbors, friends, and/or co-workers.

- Find and join a support group for people with similar health issues (your local hospital or community service agency, such as United Way, may help you connect to one in your area).

- Locate special interest groups for exercise or renewal such as cycling or hiking clubs, quilters groups, or collector's organizations.

- Keep abreast of current health issues and preventive approaches. Awareness of the consequences of not caring for yourself can, of itself, be motivational.

Education is a great motivator, for we realize what it is that we are facing and we can learn how to avoid, postpone, or overcome challenges to our health. Go online or visit your local library to learn more about the health concerns that you are facing.

Subscribe to a medically-based health newsletter such as *The Wellness Newsletter* from the University of California at Berkeley Health Science Center. Similar informative newsletters produced by medical schools such as Johns Hopkins Medicine or Harvard Medical School tend to have more helpful and unbiased medical information than do commercial magazines which are dependent upon commercial endorsements.

Be patient with yourself when you deviate from your plan, have a setback, or lose motivation. Everyone struggles on life's journey in some way. Stop and make an assessment of what is going on in your life and how you want your life's journey to be as you go forward. Visualize what it is that you want. Pray to seek God's strength and guidance for your journey. Seek help from others as needed and then work to make your vision come to life for *your* life.

Whether you take care of yourself at the encouragement of another or to avoid or deter ill health, the ultimate reason to follow a plan of self-care is because *you are worth it!* Believe in yourself, improve yourself, and develop the gifts that are within you. Who you are in all of your victorious and vulnerable humanity—the good, or even greatness, that lies within you—is a gift to the world and the source of the God-given possibilities for your life.

Develop a Supportive Network

Loneliness is one of the five major fears of growing older—outliving or separation from our family and friends. Repeatedly, researchers, counselors, pastors, and physicians report that people who have a supportive network of friends do better when facing crisis or loss than those who do not.

It is more than just casual observation that supports this. Consider these observations from a clinical study:

> In one study, for example, researchers found that people who had no friends increased their risk of death over a six-month period. In another study, those who had the most

friends over a nine-year period cut their risk of death by more than sixty percent.

Friends are also helping us live better. The famed Nurses' Health Study from Harvard Medical School found that the more friends women had, the less likely they were to develop physical impairments as they aged, and the more likely they were to be leading a joyful life. In fact, the results were so significant, the researchers concluded, that not having close friends or confidants was as detrimental to your health as smoking or carrying extra weight![43]

This is one of the reasons that senior centers in countless communities are so vital. They are a means of socialization for persons who may have lost a spouse or who live away from family or friends. The traditional view of retirement can be a mixed blessing. This is a good point to stop and ask the question, "What does it mean to be retired?" Does retirement no longer carry a traditional expectation of circumstances, age and lifestyle?

There are those who end a long-time career and whose work and accomplishments are celebrated. A school teacher, corporate executive, police officer, or veteran soldier may perhaps choose a time, or employee policies determine a time, when their employment status changes to a retired status. A party or "send-off" may be held in their honor by co-workers where gifts or plaques may be awarded. It is a time of mixed-emotion, as it is the end of one part of their life and the beginning of another. For some, the supportive network of colleagues who are encountered each day ends as final farewells are said to the workplace and connections are lost.

In other cases, unusual and yet increasingly popular in the corporate world, employees continue as "consultants." The company continues to receive the skill and wisdom of a sea-

Gary G. Kindley

soned worker while saving money by not paying benefits or having long-term commitments to an employee who is not easily terminated. There may be some reduction in compensation (typically offset by retirement income) and little job security, since consultants can be fired as easily as they were hired, but there is the continued advantage of having your workplace friends close at hand.

There are retirements that occur that are merely transitions from one career to another. Someone retiring after 30 years, who started their career at age 22, still has many years of opportunity for further employment. They move from one supportive network of co-workers and business acquaintances to another, developing new friendships while still keeping many long-established relationships.

So we return to the question, "What does it mean to be retired?" If retirement is defined by the end of one phase of life and the beginning of another, then there are scores of possibilities for a wide variety of phases along our path. I know of a gentleman who is 70 years-old who has retired four times from the same company! Each time of transition is an opportunity to continue, re-establish, or begin new networks of relationships that can bring fulfillment, enjoyment, encouragement, and companionship.

Retirement for those who own their own business is different. The hard-working, self-employed shop-owners, who quietly tape the "out of business" sign to the glass as they lock the door for the very last time, can find it more lonely. When people retire and end their daily work routine, no longer restricted by work and family obligations, they may decide to move to a new community. Many upscale, exclusive residential developments geared toward the distinctive needs of older adults, such as the many "Sun City" communities, have great appeal to the newly retired. Beautiful homes in inspiring locations with manicured golf courses, deed restricted properties, and stringent neighborhood standards (no residents under 55, no old cars parked at the curb, limited visits by screaming grandchildren) have a certain appeal.

This scenario can have a different and unexpected ending. These newly-relocated retirees realize that they miss their network of friends more than they expected. Absent co-workers, neighbors, long-time physicians, and even acquaintances such as beauticians, barbers, nurses, and grocery clerks have created a hole that is not quickly filled. Some people are less skilled than others at generating a supportive network, particularly if they tend to focus on themselves or only on a small number of family members. These are often also the parents who do not handle the "empty nest syndrome" as well as others.

Phases and changes of life each have new considerations that need to be addressed. Moving away from family and friends may create a problem if health fails or crisis comes. Having a caring network of friends through neighbors, associations, or spiritual communities reduces anxiety and brings a sense of assurance and safety. When, as a pastor and counselor, I have worked with families facing significant troubles, loss, or crisis in their life, I repeatedly hear this question that is also their affirmation: "What do people do who don't have a church family?" Take this same question and substitute "faith community," "congregation (be it synagogue or mosque)" or some other supportive community, group, or circle of friends for the word "church," and you understand that the question is really an acknowledgment of their gratitude and their need for significant relationships.

We need one another. God made us that way. People who

make friends by being a friend have grasped that wonderful truth of life. If you are feeling lonely, look beyond yourself and consider ways you can connect to others. There are likely many support groups, interest groups, volunteer organizations, and service opportunities in your community. Even small towns need volunteers at schools, libraries, hospitals, and religious organizations. By being of service or joining a group or organization, you can befriend and be befriended by others who also seek a caring relationship which is a mutual blessing and gift.

Consider starting your own interest or hobby group. Use the classified ads, online bulletin boards, or post a notice at a library, senior center or other places in your community. Book clubs, service clubs, walking clubs, exercise groups, and craft groups are all opportunities to create a network of relationships that can add love and longevity to your life. When the noon-hour strikes in Austin, Texas, a small group of employees of one large corporation put on their walking shoes, leave their cubicles and desks behind, and walk briskly along the sidewalks of a nearby park three days a week. They return in time to enjoy a light yogurt and salad lunch before resuming their duties. This simple act of networking reduces stress and improves productivity as well as motivation, recreation, and nutrition!

Introverted people may find a sense of community by internet or telephone. One "home bound" woman, whose poor health made it extremely difficult for her to leave her house, used the telephone to connect with strangers and make new friends. She made calls for political parties encouraging people to vote, was the coordinator of a telephone "prayer chain" of her church, and volunteered to make "welfare checks via telephone"—daily calls to other "home bound" folks—to insure their safety and well-being.

Networks are ultimately a chain of connections. In business or personal affairs, our interconnectedness is a mark of our humanity and our need for both interpersonal and transcendent relationships. People who have greater confidence to face the challenges of life and aging are those who receive strength and hope from knowing that someone "has their back." However or wherever you connect, when you reach out beyond yourself in the simplest of ways, you find that in giving yourself away to others, the blessing of relationship will be yours as well.

Hold a Vision for the Future

One of the reasons that great military commanders have addressed their troops on the eve of a battle is not only to encourage them, but to plant in them a vision of what they can accomplish. Throughout time, noble monarchs have painted a vision of a new day dawning when foes will be vanquished and all will dwell in peace. Such optimistic visioning empowers others to overcome fear and self-defeat, and to act to bring about their desired result. Optimistic visioning moves us from surviving to thriving and is a key component of healthy living and successful aging.

Keep in mind a visual image of what you want to become, what you want your life to become. A man I knew lost his wife when she was far too young for death to have come. They had been married a little more than ten years. After struggling with his grief for some time, he used exercise as a means of working through his feelings. I noticed a change in him, both physically and emotionally. He said that he began working out as a way of venting his grief, anger, and depression over his wife's death. Then, one day, he realized that he was not going to live alone the rest of his life. He decided that he wanted to get in shape in order to be more physically attractive to a future mate. He visualized how he wanted to be and it gave him a motivating goal for exercise, nutrition, and healthy habits.

If I envision a world where no child is hungry, hurt, alone, or afraid, I am going to strive to fulfill this vision. If I pessimistically accept that poverty is unsolvable and endemic to the human condition and that peace is not possible in my lifetime, then I will never aspire to anything greater than my small vision. Great athletes, scholars, researchers and explorers have all envisioned a victory or discovery that, when propelled forward by the power of their vision, they reached out to grasp and pull that vision into the world of reality by means of persistent determination and sheer will.

If you envision your life as one that is blossoming into something greater, it will. Imagine yourself as maturing into a better person:

- A wiser adult—one who offers the wisdom of experience
- A temperate character—a person who avoids over-indulgence and models great ethics and values
- A peaceful creature—someone who cherishes life in every form as a good steward of this world, its creatures and the created order
- A lively sojourner—a delightful companion for the journey who adds joy to the lives of those who share the trip
- A caring presence—someone in whom is found comfort, grace and acceptance
- A compassionate listener—a soul who can set aside time and their own cares and needs in order to focus on those of another

- A passionate lover—one who is willing to give themselves away in body and spirit for the sake of fervent and unconditional love

- A gracious host—one who practices the gift of hospitality and grace

- A forgiving person—one who knows that in forgiving we are pardoned and that pardon releases pain for all involved

- A joyful spirit—one who delights in life, living and relationships, both human and divine

- A loyal friend—someone upon whom another can lean for trust, self-sacrifice, commitment, and friendship

- A tender companion—a fellow sojourner who understands the power of one's presence in the life of another

- A generous heart—a selfless person who understands that it is in giving that we receive

- An inquiring mind—a thirst for knowledge and understanding of this world and all who inhabit it

- A welcoming soul—a spirit of an open heart, an open mind, and an open door to all who need God's grace

It is tough to have a sense of hope if you have no vision for your future. What encouragement and inspiration I have received from friends like Marilyn Johnson, whose vision for the future could not be restrained by life-ending illness. There are some who give-up hope when the horror of tragedy strikes. Marilyn offered her viewpoint on the aggressive cancer that was sapping the life from her body: "We all are going to die," she told me, "How we die is irrelevant; how we live is important!" Being the young pastor that I was, I wanted to write down her words of wisdom before they faded from my memory. Marilyn saw me scribbling on the back of one of my business cards and asked, "Do you need me to say it again?" We both laughed and then, ever the high school English teacher that she was, she added, "Be certain to spell 'irrelevant' with a double- r!"

Marilyn was grieved to leave her family behind and not to see her teenage son graduate from high school, but she was not without a vision that life for her family would go on and that life for her spirit would also continue. Just before Christmas, in a tradition that I had established with our church's youth ministry, teens and their sponsors would go from house to house singing Christmas carols—but with a different ending to their evening in mind. They were told that at one home, their songs of faith would lead them to the Christ child. After singing on Marilyn's front porch, we walked around to the rear of the ranch house to the barn. There in the corral, amidst bales of hay, was a young couple with a newborn baby in a traditional nativity pose. It was deeply moving as voices hushed and we sang Silent Night. That night, the Christ child was born again in our hearts behind the home of a woman who understood that life is not only about what is seen but about having a vision of things unseen.

People of faith can claim the strength of God's Spirit to help them develop and fulfill their vision of the future. Because we do not journey alone, we can claim the transcendent power that lifts us out of the mire of our woes to the mountaintops of wonder. The choices are ours, but there is a power that adds potency to our efforts

Hold a vision for your future. Live boldly. Live hopefully. Your life may have obstacles and daily struggles and limitations, but you also have possibilities. Think again of Helen Keller, Ludwig von Beethoven, and the greatness of people with seemingly insurmountable obstacles. Hold a vision for your future that is optimistic, hopeful, and rooted in the gifts and potential that you bring to life, then live and work to make your vision a reality!

What the Nine Qualities Mean for You

Don't be anxious or bemoan not having all or several of these characteristics. Strive for them! Move toward wellness and being a whole person of God by having a plan of self-care and assessing your attitude, perspective and goals.

What do you want your life to look like? What do you want to say when you near the end of your journey and look back at what your years have held? "I wished I had done this," or "If only I had done that," are not the sort of things I want to say when reflecting upon my journey.

There is no one who looks back and cannot see something that they would change, do-over, or avoid in their past. Every human journey and relationship holds things that we have done or said that we regret, or deeds or words that we felt needed to be done or we intended to speak that we never made happen. These are the things we need to surrender and leave behind.

What we carry with us is the thrill of life: enduring relationships, cherished memories, accomplished successes, celebrated joys, and sacred moments. Love never ends, never dies, never succumbs, never surrenders (unless it does so in the name of love for another), and is never forgotten.

Cope well on your journey. Consider each new day as a gift, and treasure what is sacred, giving to the wind that which is failure, regret, or misfortune. When you do, your well-being will soar and you will find yourself becoming the whole person of God you are intended to be.

For Reflection

1. What do you do for self-renewal and personal growth? What path or place leads you to a time or place of self-care (this may be a daily prayer time, a retreat location, or a favorite activity, etc.)?

2. Which of the nine coping factors are most important to you? Which do you possess?

3. Consider one characteristic of "healthy copers" that you would like to develop, and consider what you need to do to make it a reality in your life. Make a written plan or steps to accomplish your goal and begin!

LOOKING OVER
THE HILL
What Medical Science Has in Store

"A man too busy to take care of his health is like a mechanic too busy to take care of his tools."
—Spanish Proverb

"The greatest wealth is health."
—Virgil

"I drive way too fast to worry about cholesterol."
—Anonymous

For Me, It's Personal

At midnight on Thanksgiving Day 2004, at the age of eighty-eight, my mother's body died and her spirit entered into life immortal. In truth, my mother had died some time ago and I had already shed my tears at her loss. Mother had Alzheimer's disease.

Alzheimer's disease (usually abbreviated AD) has been called one of the cruelest of illnesses. It is named for the

German physician, Alois Alzheimer, who in 1906 first recognized the unique changes to the brain tissues in a woman who had died with what was described as an unusual mental illness. Though improved medical imaging or laboratory testing may soon make diagnosis in a living patient possible, AD is still only definitively diagnosed at a post-mortem examination of brain tissues. Typically, Alzheimer's is recognized through the syndrome of cognitive dysfunction and symptoms associated with it, along with family history.[44]

My aunt, the second younger sister of my mother, died with the disease some three years earlier. Another aunt, mother's immediate younger sister, died with Alzheimer's in June 2009. Of course, no one dies of Alzheimer's disease anymore than someone dies of AIDS—the Acquired Immune Deficiency Syndrome. Death comes from opportunistic and related illnesses that are brought on more quickly because of these disease processes.

Simply put, one's brain is the computer that runs the body and digests data for processing, storage, and retrieval. When the brain malfunctions, so does the body. The body becomes more susceptible to infectious disease and illness due to a slower immune response, diminished habits of hygiene, and loss of appetite. Lack of cognitive function can also lead to hazardous behavior. Some Alzheimer's patients have wandered from their homes in extreme weather and have succumbed to dehydration or hypothermia. Some have over-medicated themselves, unable to realize that they were repeatedly taking their prescribed daily medication only minutes apart. Others have died from injuries or smoke inhalation caused by accidents or fires, such as the woman who was attempting to cook with plastic containers on a gas stove.

Mother's cause of death, a urinary tract infection that led to sepsis, was hardly the heart attack or stroke which she had long feared. Her Alzheimer's disease left her less aware of her own body's symptoms, so she failed to complain until the infection was too advanced for her weakened immune system to defend.

Alzheimer's leaves tell-tale beta-amyloid plaques and tangled bundles of fibers called neurofibrillary tangles, in the brain, interfering with proper information processing and networking between neurons at the synaptic level. Neurons are similar to transistors that hold and pass along information. Tens of thousands of neurons may combine together to contain one thought or idea. The synapse is where connections are made so that communication between neurons can occur. Thus, through this highly complex neuro-chemical process, thoughts and ideas can be processed and completed. Alzheimer's disease appears to interfere with the normal chemistry and structure of the brain, causing nerve cells to die.[45]

In effect, this short-circuits both short-term and long-term memory, as well as cognitive function. As Alzheimer's begins to diminish brain function, the resulting chaos begins with forgetfulness and disassociation—mistaking a hairbrush for a razor, putting the paper towels in the refrigerator instead of the pantry—and escalates into loss of both short-term and long-term memory, inability to recognize even significant loved ones, and an inability to communicate.[46]

I realized how rapidly my mother's illness was escalating when she forgot my birthday. Mother never forgot a holiday, birthday, anniversary, or other milestone. For years, she began Christmas shopping in September, planned meticulously in advance how she was to celebrate someone's special day, and was always ahead of the curve in anticipating things that the rest of the family had yet to think about.

For some people, the disease process is rapid. Mother first forgot my birthday in December and died the following Thanksgiving. For others, years may go by with a gradual slide down a slope toward cognitive oblivion. Either way, Alzheimer's wreaks havoc on patients, significantly impacting their families, health care providers, and health care institutions themselves.

As twenty-first century people, we turn to medical science to help us better understand and cope with serious health issues that seem beyond our control. There is much research underway, and physicians and researchers are optimistic that new medication and treatments in the years ahead will make Alzheimer's a far more treatable, if not curable, disease. For assessment, there is a thirty-question Mini-Mental State Exam, sometimes called the Folstein Test, created by Marshal Folstein, M.D., Susan Folstein, M.D., and Paul McHugh, M.D. It is a brief verbal exam that can be given in under ten minutes that is 90% accurate in assessing a decline in cognitive impairment. Alzheimer's patients will drop two to four points each year.[47]

One small clinical trial using gene therapy has given promise to slowing the decline in mental functioning through such procedures. In this particular study, six patients with early-stage Alzheimer's received a gene transfer. Follow-up testing over the next twenty-two months revealed a thirty-six to fifty-one percent slowing in cognitive decline than had been seen in the fourteen months prior to the treatment. This is just one of a growing number of possible treatments as we look to the future of care and management of Alzheimer's and other forms of dementia.[48]

Wisdom from the Experts

What do experts have to tell us when the future may seem especially bleak for those of us with such a nightmarish disease in our genetic history? Out of concern for my own medical future, and in the course of research for this book, I spoke with four physicians: a gerontologist, an internist, a psychiatrist, and a world-class clinical researcher in neurology. I chose these four based upon several criteria. All are board certified in their respective fields. They trained at respected universities and medical centers representing different regions of the country, remain current with ongoing developments in their area of practice through pursuit of continuing education, and are respected by their peers.

Ronald C. Petersen, M.D., Ph D, is Professor of Neurology and Director of the Mayo Alzheimer's Disease Research Center. A world-class clinical researcher in neurology and epidemiology, particularly in the areas of aging and dementia, Dr. Petersen was a physician to President Ronald Reagan at the time of his struggle with Alzheimer's disease.

William T. Goldman, M.D. is a psychiatrist whose busy practice in the affluent community of Southlake, serves the Dallas-Fort Worth metroplex. He also is adjunct Clinical Professor at the University of Texas at Arlington, and sees a broad range of patients with a focus on diagnosis and psychopharmacology.

Paul Kim, M.D. is a sought-after gerontologist and internal medicine specialist who has treated countless patients diagnosed with Alzheimer's disease and other types of cognitive impairment. Respected by his colleagues, he has served as Chief of Staff at North Hills Medical Center in Fort Worth, Texas.

Michael Horoda, M.D. is an internist who has served in clinical practice in Dallas as well as in the field of occupational medicine, counseling his patients on the importance of preventive medicine. Here is what they have to say on the matter of growing older and the future of modern medicine.

An Interview with Ronald C. Petersen, M.D., Ph.D., Director of The Mayo Alzheimer's Disease Research Center

Dr. Ronald Petersen had just returned from a conference in Paris when we visited by phone. He is a widely sought-after speaker, and I had missed meeting with him when he was in Dallas only a few weeks prior to our conversation. He was kind to return my call and shared both his experience and concern regarding the current state of medical research pertaining to Alzheimer's and other types of cognitive impairment.

When there were signs of cognitive decline noted by President Ronald Reagan's primary physician, Dr. Petersen was called-in to examine President Reagan who, along with Nancy Reagan, had been patients of the Mayo Clinic for years. The Reagan's decision to disclose the diagnosis through the President's hand-written letter to the world raised awareness and also increased the public's questions about Alzheimer's Disease. Dr. Petersen offered this insight:

> At the time that I was working with them, both President and Mrs. Reagan were active people who strived to lead healthy lives. They had been coming to Mayo [Clinic] for their routine health care for some time. When the President's cognitive impairment was assessed during his routine exam, I was called to consult.
>
> There is currently no definitive way to diagnose Alzheimer's until post-mortem. Without a physical examination of the brain, it is not yet possible to confirm the presence of amyloid proteins, which are the signature of Alzheimer's dementia.
>
> The primary role of clinical assessment of cognitive impairment lies with the physician. Having an established relationship with a physician is a basic component of good

healthcare and helps that physician to provide a higher quality of care. Through knowledge and assessment of your medical history and familiarity with your unique situation, your primary care physician can be your best resource for better health.

I asked Dr. Petersen to elaborate about how Alzheimer's or other cognitive-impairing illness can be assessed:

> The Mini-Mental State Exam (MMSE or Folstein Test) is a crude indicator of deterioration in memory and cognition. Many factors must be taken into account. Mild cognitive impairment may or may not be a forerunner of Alzheimer's. When impairment goes beyond what we expect for normal aging, this is an alert that more serious cognitive decline may be occurring. Markers that the physician may consider include a complete physical workup with blood chemistry. When indicated, Magnetic Resonance Imaging (MRI) may be used to provide some indication of the structure of the brain including atrophy or shrinkage. A spinal tap can also be revealing and help to eliminate other possibilities.

It was clear that Dr. Petersen places a great deal of emphasis on the role of the primary care physician and providing education for them through the latest research. He continued:

> If your healthcare provider knows you, then they also can be aware of noticeable changes. They know what to look for, and what is a significant change versus a normal change of the natural process of aging. They also are likely to be better equipped at considering underlying causes of cognitive decline because they are more aware of their patient's medical history.

When I asked him what he saw on the horizon for treatment of Alzheimer's and other dementia, his thoughts also included political concerns:

> Accurate and early diagnosis means that appropriate treatment can be prescribed to slow the decline and, when possible, reverse the decline in treatable dementias.
>
> It is possible that pharmacological research may give rise to a preventive therapy. It was research that pointed to aspirin's role as a preventative of heart attacks and some strokes. What is crucial is that we "wave the red flag" to our representatives in Congress to compel them to address the looming health care crisis. As Baby Boomers age, the healthcare system will be overwhelmed to address their impending health needs. Funding research studies now is absolutely fundamental to be prepared for what is to come.
>
> I am optimistic that with continued and aggressive research, we can begin to identify underlying pathology rather than simply identifying clinical symptoms. Identifying cognitive decline and being able to do something about it must both be possible.

An Interview with William T. Goldman, M.D., Psychiatrist

Dr. Todd Goldman is a personable man with a strong handshake whose laid-back manner and full head of dark hair (compared to my "distinguished-gray" look) may initially disguise his significant experience and expertise as a mental health clinician. His young therapy dog, a black Labrador named "Booger," lies on the floor snoozing.

"He is especially good with children and compassionate when someone is crying," Dr. Goldman says of the dog. "He senses when people are hurting and wants to comfort them."

Given that there is a history of Alzheimer's and dementia in my family, I wanted to know how Dr. Goldman dealt with patients who have such a history. I asked him if there was anything that could be done to avoid being another victim, or any way that it could be determined whether or not someone was going to have the disease. Here are his thoughts:

I tell my patients not to lose sleep worrying about possibly having Alzheimer's disease. First, there is currently no test approved to accurately predict whether or not you will develop Alzheimer's, although research is underway involving use of brain scanning technology. Secondly, medication is available now and new drugs are being developed that slow the advancement of the disease in persons diagnosed with significant cognitive decline. With ongoing research, by the time it is ever a genuine concern for people who are now in their fifties, there could quite likely be drugs on the market to significantly impede its effects. Developments in preventive treatment perhaps could one day stop it in its tracks.

Exercise and a healthy diet are always essential to maintaining mental health. Your body is an intricate chemistry set with an amazing circulatory system. If you keep it in balance and avoid things which impede adequate circulation you will also be acting intentionally to promote healthy brain function. Generally speaking, maintain your cholesterol levels, keep an eye on your blood pressure, and exercise regularly for good cardiovascular health

Omega-3 fatty acids found in fish oils have been proven to promote healthy circulation, and that includes circulation in the brain. There are studies linking some non-steroidal anti-inflammatory drugs (NSAID's), such as ibuprofen, with a slowing in plaque development in the brain, but the research is still ongoing and it is too soon to draw universal and definitive conclusions. Just like Aricept and other drugs specifically designed to slow Alzheimer's, there are side-effects. Each person's health should be carefully evaluated by a physician before taking daily doses of NSAID's or other medications.

I know that diet and exercise are an important part of healthy living, but keeping the brain healthy seems more of a mystery. Recalling the memorization work I once did in public school, it seemed a reflection of the educational philosophy at the time that the brain was a muscle and we needed to work it to keep it strong. In the ninth grade, I moaned and wondered why we needed to memorize the periodic table in chemistry when we could have looked it up in a book (or now online) whenever we needed it! Dr. Goldman confirmed that our teachers were correct; the brain is a use-it-or-lose-it organ of the body and the more we use it the greater chance we have of brain health. He continued:

> It is certain that keeping active and mentally alert is always a positive thing. People's attitudes, activity levels, socialization, and intellectual stimulation all contribute to cognitive health. People in their seventies, eighties, and nineties who play scrabble, read books, work crossword puzzles, and perform other mentally challenging activities will do better at maintaining cognitive function than those who don't. It really is a use-it-or-lose-it prescription. I would also add that watching television does not count as mental exercise!
>
> There are good things on the horizon regarding improving mental health. There already is better treatment for depression through pharmacology, and there's the genuine possibility of more effective remedies to delay onset of Alzheimer's, or perhaps even stop or reverse its effects. Better management of bipolar and other disorders will be developed through research. Improved availability of mental healthcare is essential as the demand increases due

to the extended longevity of the growing population. This will require greater insurance coverage and greater funding for mental healthcare. These are two critical issues that must be addressed.[49]

I think that optimism is important. It is true that about one in two persons in their eighties and nineties will develop some form of dementia such as Alzheimer's. That also means that one in two will not. Now is the time to focus on what we can do to better care for ourselves so that it is more likely that we can be one of the fifty-percent who remain healthy, and even shift the balance of percentages in favor of avoiding the disease altogether.

I jumped-in at this point and asked, "I agree that an attitude of optimism improves a great many things in life, but are there dementias that we can actually cure?"

Some types of cognitive decline are reversible. For example, dementia that is caused by vitamin deficiency, medication-induced dementia, and pseudo-dementia caused by depression can be effectively treated. Approximately fifteen percent of patients presenting for workup of dementia have a reversible dementia.

An Interview with Paul Kim, M.D., Gerontologist

Dr. Paul Kim is another more-experienced-than-his-youthful-looks-reveals medical professional whose practice has grown so rapidly that he stopped accepting new patients for a time. We met at a restaurant as he took a break from a continuing education event he was attending. I asked him what he thought we would see as the greatest leap forward in medicine regarding issues of aging and physical/mental health in the next decade. His response was encouraging:

There is real hope that the greatest leap forward in the next decade regarding aging and mental health will be in the field of Alzheimer's Syndrome. Currently, we have several medications available. Unfortunately, none of the current treatments are cures. Alzheimer's can affect one out of ten patients over the age of sixty-five, and up to half of patients above eighty years of age. I see the enormous burden it puts on families with regard to a patient's change in behavior, the financial impact of adequate care, and the mental stress on care givers and other loved ones. Hopefully we will see medicines that significantly slow down or even cure the disease process. The current treatments are better than placebo, but not great.

Not wanting to be too narrowly focused on the possibilities for the future, I shifted our conversation to check-out the current state of health care. I asked what he considered to be significant accomplishments of science and medicine regarding aging and health during his years of practice as a physician and gerontologist?

This question seems to depend upon which specialist you speak with. No doubt there have been tremendous advances in cardiovascular medicine. The use of stents, less invasive techniques, and new medications has reduced cardiac-related deaths. The new techniques reduce recovery time for patients and carry fewer risks of complications. Advances in how surgeries and procedures are performed make the methods of a decade ago seem archaic.

We have better guidelines for preventive medicine, as well as better treatment for diseases. There have also been significant advances in the research and treatment of cancer, hypertension, diabetes, high cholesterol, osteoporosis, and other disease. Ten years ago we only had calcium and hormones for treatment of osteoporosis. Now we have medications to reduce fracture risk and build bone quality. If a vertebral compression fracture develops, we now have procedures to treat the pain. Chemotherapy regimens for certain cancers have improved the quality of life for many patients. With continued advances, we can offer hope to many persons who are afflicted with illnesses that were untreatable in our lifetime.

It is amazing how much change has taken place in ten years. It teaches us how important it is to keep learning, and for physicians to keep up with the advances as they occur.

Both Dr. Petersen and Dr. Goldman had mentioned that there are various types of dementia, but had not actually differentiated them, so I asked Dr. Kim how Alzheimer's Syndrome was unique. Then I did what you would have done if you were sitting across from a gerontologist and wanted to know a scientific answer to our common plight; I asked the question: Why do we age?

Alzheimer's disease is a slow progressive loss of brain cells which results in memory loss, inability to perform activities of daily living, loss of language, and inability to learn new tasks. It also results in personality and behavior changes. Alzheimer's effects 4.5 million Americans—one in ten of people over sixty-five and one in two of people over eighty-five. It accounts for sixty to seventy percent of dementia cases.

There are other forms of dementia, which include pressure hydrocephalus, vascular dementia, Parkinson's dementia, as well as less common forms. Early consultation with a physician and diagnosis is your greatest advantage. Typical pressure hydrocephalus may have a surgical cure, and medication currently available may slow down the disease and stabilize symptoms. Continued research is underway to find a cure.

We age because our DNA continues to replicate itself, and much like making a copy of a copy of a copy, changes occur. Studies have shown that genes may become defective over time. Aging is [the process of] our cells dying faster than they are being replaced, or having less function. There are many theories on aging. We need to maximize our physical, emotional, and spiritual self and be blessed with good genes to live a long life.

An Interview with Michael Horoda, M.D., Internist

The irony was not lost on me that I was sitting in a Mexican restaurant eating refried beans and tortilla chips that had likely been cooked in hydrogenated oils while interviewing a physician on nutrition and preventive medicine! Dr. Michael Horoda, (pronounced ho-RO-duh), is passionate about healthcare and music—he has a small recording studio at his home. Still in his forties, he emphasizes to his patients the importance of good nutrition and strives to practice what he prescribes. Even so, he is not an "eat-only-twigs-and-spring-water" sort of guy, as he enjoys gourmet cooking along with his music. I asked what guidance he gave his patients regarding the use vitamins and other nutritional supplements. Here are his comments, followed by a list of supplements he recommends and why:

> Supplements help to replace those important elements of our diet where we are deficient. Diet, not medication or supplements, is the starting place for health. For example, persons deficient in magnesium should incorporate whole grains, seafood, and nuts into their diet. Protein is especially essential as people advance in age.

Dr. Horoda next shared something that surprised me, Medicare covers some diagnostic blood tests that can be prescribed to determine what supplements a patient needs according to their personal body chemistry. For geriatric patients, this can be a much more precise means of helping them to select supplements rather than simply taking whatever is suggested by the latest issue of their favorite magazine.

Your physician should be consulted whenever you add or change the use of nutritional supplements, and this is especially critical for people with pre-existing health conditions or who take other medication that may be contraindicated with the use of certain supplements. The key nutritional supplements that Dr. Horoda recommends for many of his patients who are age 55 and over include:

- Bromaline: a pineapple extract that aids in the digestion of protein.

- B-complex vitamins: The B-complex vitamins are actually a group of eight vitamins, which include thiamine (B1), riboflavin (B2), niacin (B3), pyridoxine (B6), folic acid (B9), cyanocobalamin (B12), pantothenic acid and biotin. These vitamins are essential for the breakdown of carbohydrates into glucose to provide energy for the body, and the breakdown of fats and proteins which aids the normal functioning of the nervous system.

- L-Cystiene and L-Glutathion—essential amino acids that are basic building blocks of health.

- Vitamin E (400 i.u.): an antioxidant and immune modulator found in whole grains and nuts.

- Zinc (50 mg.): helps to maintain a healthy immune system, is needed for the synthesis of DNA, and helps to improve the integrity of skin to aid in wound healing.

- Glucosamine: helps to preserve mobility and has been shown, in some cases, to slow or even reverse progressive osteoarthritis.

- Vitamin C (Ascorbic Acid, 500 mg. twice daily)—helps to produce collagen, a protein needed for healthy bones, cartilage, and vertebral discs.

Michael Horoda speaks with the passion of a man who knows that he can help improve people's lives and a sense of urgency in wanting to do so. I inquired about his expectations of what the future would hold for medical advances:

There are exciting things happening now which hold real promise for future possibilities; such as the use of stem cells. In one case, a patient's jaw had to be surgically removed because of a neoplasm of the mouth. A titanium cage was made in the shape of his jaw, seeded with stem cells, and then implanted in his shoulder. His own body acted as an incubator for the process. New bone formed and was replanted to replace his jaw. Such a procedure was unheard of before the use of stem cells.

There is the use of collagen matrix to replace the tips of noses damaged by injury or cancer. There continue to be better immunosuppressant drugs to overcome organ transplant rejection. The use of inhaled insulin, a drug previously requiring injections, can allow patients freedom from frequent needle sticks. These are just some of the new and exciting things that are opening windows of opportunity for healing and medical advances.

I especially appreciate that he urges his patients to be wise consumers of medical care. There are medical tests that we do not need as often as they have historically been administered, and ones that we should receive and should insist upon if they are not prescribed.

Unless there is a family or personal medical history of cardiovascular disease, you only need an EKG (also known as ECG or electro-cardiogram) about once every five years. Some guidelines still call for them annually, but this usually is not necessary. An EKG is an electrical snapshot of the heart from twelve different views. It gives a good baseline so that your physician can note changes in your heart's electrical system. Remember that you can have a regular pulse but an abnormal EKG.

An echocardiogram is another good tool for keeping vigilant of your heart health. Dependent upon your personal or family medical history, one should be taken between ages fifty-five to sixty-five in order to establish a baseline for your heart's anatomy. An echocardiogram can detect subtle abnormalities or enlargement. It is an essential tool for patients with a heart murmur or a history of arrhythmia or hypertension.

Just as you should know your blood pressure numbers, you should also know your Body Mass Index (BMI). It is a good diagnostic tool to assess obesity, malnutrition, and hydration.

As our lunch discussion ended and we stood to leave, Dr. Horoda made a statement that I take with me. He said, "I am reminded of a quote I saw in a colleague's office: 'Be careful to take care of your body. Where else are you going to live?'

"No, I Won't Go!"

Unlike any time before in human history, we live in an age of preventable, treatable, and even curable illness. We have heard what the experts tell us that we need to do in order to live healthier, happier lives. So why do so many people—and there are more than you may imagine—not seek health care or practice basic self-care?

According to Prevention of Chronic Disease, an online serial publication, the State of Georgia conducted a cancer awareness and education campaign. Some results that came from that program and study included why people do not seek medical care to screen for treatable or preventable illness. Here are the most common responses:

- I just don't.
- Too embarrassed.
- I don't have the time.
- Can't afford it and I don't have insurance.
- I'm not that old.
- I'll go to a doctor when I'm really sick.

In contrast, the most common reasons why people specifically sought out cancer screening were:

- They wanted to be certain that they didn't have cancer.
- They knew you should be screened.
- They had a family history of cancer.[50]

Real Men Get Check-Ups

When we understand the consequence of illness and our action or inaction in preventing it, there seems to be a somewhat greater willingness to seek help or to make changes in our life-style. When we actually encounter illness and its consequence for our daily manner of living, we are even more likely to take action to regain what we have lost, or might lose, to illness and the disease process.

Since men tend to be especially reluctant to seek health care, particularly wellness care, here is some information important for men to know and take to heart. To provide greater motivation for guys out there, I will begin with health concerns more closely related to sexual performance.

- *Prostate cancer* is the most commonly occurring cancer in men, excluding skin cancer, and the second leading cause of cancer-related death for American men. It is also quite treatable when detected early. A blood test (PSA) or urine test (PCA3) and a digital rectal exam are essential for early detection.[51] The prostate is a small organ anterior to the rectum that produces most of the fluid in ejaculate. It commonly enlarges as men age, and medication or surgery may be required when the swelling affects urination.

- *Testicular cancer* can be detected early through self-exams and usually occurs in men ages fifteen to thirty-five. It is the leading cause of cancer in men ages twenty to thirty-four[52]. Testicular cancer is increasing among young men in many countries, including the U.S., according to the American Cancer Society (ACS). About 8,000 men will be diagnosed and 390 will die of the disease this year, the ACS estimates. Testicular cancer is highly curable. More than nine out of ten men with testicular cancer are diagnosed with a small, localized tumor that is highly treatable. Even if the cancer has spread at diagnosis, many men with testicular cancer are treated successfully and have an excellent chance of survival, with Lance Armstrong being a famous example.[53]

- *Diabetes* is a disease affecting the body's ability to manage blood sugar which raises your risk of heart attack and stroke. It can also lead to "unpredictability" in sexual performance in some men as it may contribute to erectile dysfunction.

- *Smoking* and *increased blood cholesterol* impedes circulation that is vital for all organs to function properly, and yes, men, I do mean *all* organs.

- *Colo-rectal cancer* screening can be done in a "two-for-one" exam. While receiving a digital exam for your prostate check-up, you can be screened for colon cancer through a simple test (no invasive scope involved) to detect intestinal bleeding. Your physician, after checking your prostate, wipes a minute amount of fecal material from the exam glove across a special pad that can detect blood—a possible indicator of colon cancer. This does not replace the more thorough sigmoidoscopy/colonoscopy that most physicians recommend should be conducted every three to five years after age forty-nine.

You wouldn't consider spending $40,000 on a vehicle and then not changing the oil until the engine is damaged. Avoiding or postponing annual wellness exams can allow disease time to spread and advance, costing you much more physically, emotionally, and financially. The impact on your family for the treatment of major disease or cancer can be avoided through simple screenings and annual physical exams.

If you have medical insurance, many insurance companies pay for an annual wellness exam in order to reduce their cost of paying for treatment of advanced disease. If you don't have insurance, but have a moderate income, I received a thorough physical exam with blood tests for not much more than the price of two rounds of golf at a nice course. If you have limited financial resources and no insurance, most county hospitals or county health centers have out-patient clinics where you can schedule routine wellness care. Government-funded healthcare also appreciates the advantage of wellness care and early detection to avoid the burden of expensive treatments on taxpayers.

Recommended Schedule of Health Screenings[54]

Table 1 – General Adult Screenings

Screening	Purpose	20-29	30-39	40-49	50-59	60+
Cholesterol and HDL-C	Identify people at risk for high coronary artery disease	Every 5 years depending upon level	Every 5 years depending upon level	Every 1-3 years depending upon level	Annually	Annually
EKG	Identify injury to heart or irregular rhythms			Baseline test between ages 40-45	Annually	Annually
General Physical Exam	Detects conditions before symptoms develop	Every 2-3 years	Every 2-3 years	Every 2-3 years	Annually	Annually
Immunizations	Create immunity against a particular disease	Tetanus/Diphtheria/Pertussis – 1 dose then Tetanus/D booster every 10 years. Measles-Mumps-Rubella 1 or 2 doses. Influenza annually age 50 and older. Pneumococcal vaccine once after age 65. Hepatitis A& B (adults at risk). Varicella (chickenpox) 2 doses. Herpes Zoster (shingles) once after 60. HPV-3 doses (19-26yo females). Meningococcal-1 or more doses if at risk				
Rectal Exam	Detect abnormalities in the rectum				Annually	Annually

Flexible Sigmoidoscopy/ Colonoscopy	Detect cancers and polyps on the inside wall of the colon before they become cancerous				Every 3-5 years	Every 3-5 years
Hemoccult	Detect blood in stool to screen for various diseases				Annually	Annually
Tonometry	Screen for Glaucoma	Annually	Every 2 years after age 35	Every 2 years	Every 1-2 years	Annually
Breast self-exam	Look for color changes, skin irregu- larities, lumps, and changes in the nipples	Monthly	Monthly	Monthly	Monthly	Monthly

Bone Density	Detect osteoporosis (the loss of bone mass which can increase risk of fractures)			Baseline at menopause for women, and at age 60 in men, particularly if there is a family history of osteoporosis. Repeat measurements depending upon results and physician's advice.
Fasting Glucose Test	Detect diabetes, pre-diabetes, other illnesses	If overweight and other risk factors for diabetes are identified	If overweight and other risk factors for diabetes are identified	Age 45 and above, every three years or upon the advice of a physician

Table 2 – Women's Health Screenings

Screening	Purpose	20-29	30-39	40-49	50-59	60+
Mammography	Detect cancer and precancerous changes		Baseline test between ages 35-40	Every 1-2 years	Annually	Annually
Pap Smear	Detect abnormal cells that may become cancerous	Annually	Annually	Annually	Annually	Annually

Pelvic Exam	Detect cancer and pre-cancerous changes of the cervix	Annually	Annually	Annually	Annually	Annually

Table 3 – Men's Health Screenings

Screening	Purpose	20-29	30-39	40-49	50-59	60+
Prostate Specific Antigen	Detect prostate cancer in the earliest stages			Annually after age 40	Annually	Annually
Digital rectal exam	Identify enlargement of or tumor in the prostate gland			Annually after age 40	Annually	Annually

Staying healthy and aging well is not as hard as it seems if we do the most basic things that doctors and our mothers have been telling us for decades: exercise, eat right, and stop smoking. Avoiding excess fats and sugars, drinking plenty of water, and limiting alcohol intake will all pay-off in both quality and longevity of life. A diet of antioxidant-rich foods (see addendum) maintains good circulation by promoting healthy blood vessels. Fatty foods directly attack the walls of blood vessels by depositing plaque that builds up and diminishes blood flow. Simple things such as monitoring our blood pressure, taking a vision exam, having our blood sugar tested, and doing self-exams for breast or testicular cancer can have dramatic results in improving our health. There can be payoffs to a healthy lifestyle in other ways. Cardiovascular disease can also contribute to erectile dysfunction (ED), which can have other causes as well.[55] Perhaps such knowledge will help us to be motivated to maintain healthy habits.

Your health is your own and the choice is yours. Remember that your health can also have a tremendous impact upon the lives of those around you. Lost days of work due to complications from late-detection of problems can take their toll. The emotional strain on family and friends because you waited until it was almost "too late," or even worse, waiting until it was too late to be effectively treated, can be devastating. Take care of yourself and enjoy the well-being God intended for you to experience throughout your many years of life's journey.

For Reflection

1. What medical recommendations do you need to more seriously consider in order to take better care of yourself? What do you need to do differently or start doing that you have hesitated or refused to do?

2. How much do you depend upon medical science to aid you in your pursuit of successful aging? How do you weigh the balance between "naturally" aging and using medical science to prolong life?

3. Have you discussed with loved ones your preferences regarding life-sustaining measures should your health fail but your body has not died? What role does quality of life play in your discussion? What role does faith play in your discussion?

CHECKING-OUT THE WILDFLOWERS

Alternative Approaches to Health and Well-Being

"Medicine provides the means to treat diseases. Knowledge is the foundation of good health."

—Eric J. Lien, PhD.

"Life expectancy would grow by leaps and bounds if green vegetables smelled as good as bacon."

—Doug Larson

"If I'd known I was gonna live this long, I'd of taken better care of myself."

—Eubie Blake, on reaching the age of 100

Complementary and Alternative Medicine

It is difficult to break certain habits, particularly certain habitual ways of thinking. You might find it unusual, or even antithetical, for me to follow an interview of four medical doctors with a chapter on alternative medicine. In truth, well-being can embrace many different approaches. Traditional or allopathic medicine and alternative or integrative medical approaches can combine to enhance each other by offering the best they have. Today, this approach is referred to by the National Institutes of Health as *complementary and alternative medicine* or CAM.

According to the University of California—San Francisco School of Medicine:

> "CAM is defined as the 'broad range of healing philosophies, approaches, and therapies that mainstream Western (conventional) medicine does not commonly use, accept, study, understand, or make available.' CAM therapies may be used alone, as an alternative to conventional therapies, or in addition to conventional, mainstream medicine to treat conditions and promote wellbeing."[56]

Since the mid-1990's, the University of Texas Southwestern Medical School, one of the premier medical schools in the nation, known for their cutting-edge medical research, has included integrative medicine as a part of their curriculum. Ironically, the program which started as panel discussions about alternative medicine was funded by a research foundation established by the woman who pioneered yoga instruction in Dallas.[57]

There are times when surgery is essential to save a life, such as cases of physical trauma, a ruptured appendix, or encapsulated tumors that can be successfully removed and a cancer cured. There are times when invasive procedures can be avoided through other approaches to health that are just as, or even more, successful and without the complication or side-effects from surgical intervention.

As someone who has more than a little experience with

traditional medicine, I commend the many different philosophies, disciplines, and approaches that contribute to wholeness of body, mind, and spirit. My journey in the discipline of medical science has taken many different and scenic paths. I share it with you now in order to place in context what is to follow, particularly for those who more easily dismiss acceptance of alternative medical practice.

I was working toward a BSN degree in Emergency Medicine after completing my undergraduate degree in Education and Psychology and just prior to ultimately entering seminary. You might say that it took me a while to determine what I wanted to do—or perhaps to respond to a calling of what I was led to do—to best use my gifts.

I worked for four years in a hospital emergency department as a Registered Emergency Medical Technician, following my undergraduate degree and during my first years in seminary. While in seminary, I spent almost a year in clinical training as a hospital chaplain at Harris Methodist Hospital in Fort Worth. Harris Methodist, a Texas Health Resources hospital, is a regional medical center, Level One Trauma Center, and listed as one of the best hospitals in the country. I also served six years as a volunteer hospital chaplain and chaplaincy coordinator for Harris Methodist Northwest Hospital, while a parish minister in that community.

Clinical training for chaplains is not simply a spiritual experience; it challenges you intrapersonally, interpersonally, and deepens your understanding of the wonder, weakness, frustration, and frontier of medical science. Observing coronary bypass and other surgery, serving as a member of a medical emergency response team ("Dr. Heart/Code Blue"), entering into dialogue with physicians and nurses, and other clinical experiences are a part of hospital chaplaincy training.

With this much experience in clinical, traditional medical settings, some would find it unusual that I would also embrace many different alternative approaches. In 1992, my youngest son, John, was born robust and healthy with the help of alternative medicine. During her third trimester of pregnancy, his mother slipped and fell in the shower injuring her back. We learned that there was little that traditional medical science could do to help. X-rays were out of the question and prescription drugs for pain carried the risk of side-effects for both she and our baby. At the urging of a friend, Liz went to a Chinese Medical Practitioner and received acupuncture treatments. To our amazement, they were even covered by our health insurance! I later learned that the American Medical Association acknowledges the medical benefit of acupuncture for the relief of pain and many inflammatory diseases, though I am told that the AMA has noted that the science of *why* it works is still unclear and puzzling for some.

When I had a bulging cervical disk that was impinging upon a nerve in my spine, the pain led me to see my physician who referred me to a neurosurgeon. Following scans and X-rays, I was scheduled for a laminectomy on the Monday after Easter, a little more than six weeks away. This procedure removes the spongy material that protrudes from the disc, the cause of pain from the resulting nerve compression. I was in pain and did not wish to be heavily medicated, lest that I would be impeded from my duties, so I tried a series of acupuncture treatments while awaiting surgery. The week prior to my surgery, scans were repeated and the neurosurgeon said that there was no reason to proceed with the surgery. The protruding disk material had been reabsorbed, the inflammation diminished, and I was no longer in pain. I had expected acupuncture to help relieve my pain, but I did not anticipate it helping me to avoid surgery altogether.

In my move back to the Dallas/Fort Worth area, after serving churches for a decade in the Central Texas region, I injured my back. I had tried anti-inflammatory medication, but it only seemed to upset my stomach more than it reduced the pain. I learned of Ronald Blaha, D.C., C.C.S.P., C.A.C., a Dallas chiropractor who is also credentialed in chiropractic sports medicine as well as acupuncture. Dr. Blaha shatters the absurd stereotype of chiropractic medicine as simply the practice of "getting your back popped." Well beyond that and even beyond the practice of some chiropractors, he did not simply "adjust" a portion of the spine to correct vertebral sublaxation, but considered the condition of the whole body.

He gave me a general physical examination, which was very similar to the annual exams I had received from my medical doctors through the years. He examined blood pressure, pulse, lungs, reflexes, eyes, ears, mouth, and skin. He examined all of my joints, testing range of motion—which no other physician had ever done. All-in-all, my skeptical, empirical attitude found new respect for this systematic, thorough, and scientific healer and his practice of chiropractic medicine. Following x-rays of my spine, a follow-up visit was scheduled to review all of the findings. My symptoms and x-rays had indicated the need for an MRI (magnetic resonance imaging), so that procedure was scheduled. The results led to a diagnosis of a bulging disc, a congenital fusion of two vertebrae—something many previous physicians had not mentioned following similar x-rays—scoliosis, and osteoporosis. The protrusion from the disc was the primary cause of my pain and the tingling in my arm.

Without anti-inflammatory medication and within a matter of two weeks of chiropractic treatment, I was feeling much better. In six weeks, my symptoms were almost totally gone, and by eight weeks from my first treatment, I was completely free of tingling, pain, and discomfort. I resumed my regular work-outs at the gym, after a period of much lighter physical therapy. I was a believer in the benefit of capable and experienced chiropractic care.

As I explored the benefits of CAM, I interviewed practitioners of chiropractic, acupuncture, homeopathic therapy, and yoga.

An Interview with Colin Tkachuk, D.C.

Dr. Colin Tkachuk (pronounced kuh-chuk'), has a background as a registered nurse supervising a cardio-thoracic care unit at a large hospital. The appeal of chiropractic care's focus on wellness lured him from allopathic medicine to completing chiropractic school. He moved from Canada to Texas, and opened his practice in the affluent and quasi-bucolic town of Colleyville, one of many suburban enclaves in the Dallas/Fort Worth metroplex.

Given that he has worked in traditional medicine and is now a chiropractic physician, I asked him his perspective on how alternative medicine impacts aging and health. He made an interesting observation regarding the new consumerism and healthcare choices:

> The 'baby boomer generation' is more aware of choices in health care and they are willing to look for alternatives beyond allopathic medicine. We are beyond the days of "I must do whatever the doctor says!" Many people take seri-

ously the role of being a wise consumer of health care options. They research prescriptions they receive from their medical doctor and decide if they wish to have them filled. We are moving beyond the day when taking supplements was considered alternative medicine and having your chest cut open was considered mainstream health care.

There is also a paradigm shift that places focus on wellness and prevention rather than the treatment of illness and disease. Economically, it makes more sense to spend a dollar on wellness versus ten dollars on hospitalization and surgery.

Chiropractic medicine has become more widely accepted than merely a treatment for back and neck pain. Chiropractic improves nervous system function and addresses pediatric health, immune disorders, and inflammatory disease. There are more chiropractic schools than ever before, with thirteen in the United States and also schools in Europe.

As I did with the medical doctors in the previous interviews, I wanted to know some specifics that made alternative medicine a wise choice. I asked Dr. Tkachuk for an example of an illness or disease process that is best helped by chiropractic medicine, and what was on the horizon for chiropractic care.

One of the most common diseases of adults is osteoarthritis. Chiropractic adjustments keep the joints moving, reducing stiffness and promoting flexibility with a healthy range of motion. Motion is life and chiropractic medicine helps keep people moving.

An Interview with Karim Harati-Zadeh, DC, FIAMA, FASA

Dr. Harati-Zadeh is a Fellow of the Acupuncture Society of America, a Fellow of the International Academy of Medical Acupuncture, and is certified by National Board of Chiropractic

Examiners and American Society of Acupuncture. He first opened his practice in Chicago and has practiced in Dallas for almost four years. His use of acupuncture for facial toning and wrinkle reduction (acupuncture stimulates the formation of collagen and relaxes facial muscles) has made him quite popular among Dallas elite, and he has been featured in *D Magazine* and *The Dallas Morning News*.

I asked him to start with "the basics." How does acupuncture work? Here is Dr. Harati-Zadeh's explanation:

> Acupuncture is one of the oldest and most commonly used systems of healing in the world, having been practiced for over 3,500 years. It has been recognized by the World Health Organization as effective in the treatment of nearly four dozen common ailments. In 1997, the National Institutes of Health found that acupuncture could be useful by itself or in combination with other therapies to treat addiction, pain, postoperative and chemotherapy nausea, nausea from pregnancy, as well as inflammatory illnesses including osteoarthritis and carpal tunnel syndrome.
>
> Through the use of strategically placed, one-time-use, sterile micro-needles, about the diameter of a human hair, the body's energy or chi (pronounced *chee*) is balanced through twelve meridians. A new procedure called electromeridian imaging, or EMI, picks up electromagnetic frequencies to allow more accurate balancing of the body's chi.
>
> Some meridians stimulate or tonify, some sedate or calm, while others balance or connect. The effectiveness has been documented in numerous scientific studies, including a European study that demonstrated the effectiveness of acupuncture as one approach to infertility. Acupuncture increases blood flow to the uterus and decreases anxiety, and stress has been shown to contribute to infertility. Depending upon the condition, typically fourteen to sixteen sessions one to three times per week are common.

Gary G. Kindley

Yoga: An Interview with Vicki Johnson, MS, RYT, LCDC

Yoga, the five-thousand-year-old eastern practice of body poses and stretches for strength, meditation, health, and relaxation, has grown in the number of westerners who practice this ancient exercise. Some may consider it just another form of physical exercise, such as running or weight-lifting; I include it here because of its direct link to improved overall health and its association with complementary integrative medicine. According to a recent study, more than 16.5 million people participate in the discipline, and 2.95 billion is spent each year on classes and props. When body, mind, and spirit are brought together through this time-honored discipline; the person moves toward wholeness and peace. Blood pressure lowers, muscles relax, stress fades, and thoughts become focused.[58]

Yoga is not a practice solely for the fit. It can also be adapted for older persons and for obese people, as well. Poses can be adjusted according to body size and physical ability, and "chair yoga" can be used for seniors.[59]

Vicki Johnson is a registered yoga teacher who teaches in Dallas and leads seminars around the nation. She has been teaching yoga since 1979 and is also a licensed chemical dependency counselor, incorporating yoga to enhance the twelve-step recovery process. I asked her for a bit of recent history to explain yoga's rise in popularity. She was ready with a response:

> People are discovering how effective yoga is for integrating body, mind, and breath. Yoga addresses so many physical and emotional issues. Back in the 1970's, community colleges, the YWCA, YMCA, and city recreation/park boards started offering yoga. Some organizations brought in skilled practitioners who were from India in order to

better understand the basic philosophy, techniques, and practice. Now many hospitals offer classes for both their staff and their community and there are classes hosted in churches and synagogues around the country.

When yoga's popularity was starting to soar, one large church-affiliated hospital, fearful of Christians thinking of yoga as another religion, asked if I would offer classes for their staff, but would call it something else. I told them, "No, it's yoga!"

Yoga reduces stress and anxiety, improves breathing, addresses muscular and alignment issues, and positively impacts the nervous system, circulatory system, and endocrine system. Yoga leads to deep and integrative healing of body, mind, and spirit.

I confess that I was in a playful mood at the time, but being a lover of stories, I asked her if she had any about someone not embracing the concept of yoga or trying it and getting stuck in a particular posture. Instead, she gave me a great example of how yoga had contributed to someone's health and changed someone's life.

There was one client who was a retired, "Type A" personality. Retirement did not suit her well and her anxiety accelerated to the point that she sought the care of a psychiatrist. He gave her some medication and referred her to me. She had some physical impairment, so we focused on individual sessions at first. After nine months, she began participating in group sessions and is like a new person. Her anxiety is reduced, her physical health has improved, and her overall attitude and outlook are remarkable.

It has also been gratifying to see the role that yoga has in the twelve-step process. As a counselor who works with people suffering chemical dependency, I have seen firsthand how effective yoga can be to reduce anxiety and improve focus and self-discipline.

Homeopathy: An Interview with Alphie Wishart, Lay Homeopath

After speaking with several people who find complementary and alternative medicine preferable to allopathic medicine, I explored the practice of homeopathy. There are many highly trained and experienced lay homeopaths and also physicians (M.D.s and D.O.s) who practice homeopathy. In the course of writing this book, I learned that there are two such physicians in Dallas, both of whom are medical doctors.

Mr. Alphie Wishart is a lay homeopath whose experience and knowledge I sought when researching the origin and practice of homeopathy. Though not a medical doctor, he is an experienced practitioner, who shared with me his background and homeopathy's history:

> Homeopathy is an empirically-based medical art, founded by Samuel Hahnemann, M.D. (1755–1843) in 1790. Hahnemann was studying the effects of Cinchona bark in order to establish a scientifically verifiable method that would reveal why Cinchona bark would cure malaria (the active principle in Cinchona bark is quinine, now famous for its anti-malarial properties). After taking regular doses of a Cinchona bark preparation and making copious clinical observations on himself, he found that the symptoms produced by taking the bark were the same symptoms of the illness, malaria. This was a clear demonstration of the principle "like cures like," which was first established by Hippocrates some 2,500 years previously. "Like cures like" simply means that medication which causes certain symptoms in a healthy person will cure those symptoms in the sick.
>
> Though homeopathy is rooted in scientific principles, it is also an art given that we have literally thousands of remedies at our disposal and each person's case is unique to that individual.

When I heard him describe it as an art, I was reminded of the term, "the *practice* of medicine." The "healing arts" are a combination of objective and subjective principles which are affected by a patient's emotional state, physical condition, and acceptance of the prescribed treatment involved. This is why pharmaceutical companies conduct blind tests that include a placebo to assure that a patient is not imagining a symptom or cure. How does a homeopath assess a patient to prescribe a treatment? Wishart explains this intriguingly unique and yet familiar tactic:

> A homeopath, in order to get at all the distinguishing features of a case, begins with what is typically a two-hour interview. This interview explores not only the details of the chief complaint, but also medical and family history while assessing lifestyle, habits, hobbies, as well as the individual's physical, mental, and emotional status. For example, if someone is diagnosed with bronchitis in conventional medicine, there are perhaps half-a-dozen antibiotics to choose from, plus some supportive therapies. That same person, being treated with homeopathy, would be individuated by the quality of the cough, other respiratory symptoms, modifying factors such as time of day, temperature, exposure, and so on. In addition, their mental emotional state would be considered, possible causes, personal and family history, and so on until the full picture was obtained. This is why, with homeopathy, ten people with a conventional diagnosis of bronchitis are each likely to receive a different remedy, since the remedy is based on the individual and not on a broad, standard diagnosis.
>
> The individuating symptoms include personality factors. One person may have feelings of enmity or intolerance, another might feel like a victim, or yet another may feel panicky. The mental and emotional state is very important in selecting the proper remedy. This includes assessing the individual's ability to process emotions, their

self-image, and their history of emotional trauma or mental health. Then we add to this the details of the physical condition and the family history. There are a multitude of factors that go into the selection of a remedy. Even though every phase of homeopathy is guided by scientifically sound and empirically-based principles, for the selection of a remedy, homeopathy requires an artful hand.

At this point, as I had done in previous interviews, I asked once more about the actual curative ability of a given treatment. I believe that any medical practice, whether a Western allopathic approach or complementary alternative medicine, is ultimately measured by its ability to cure an ailment or at least to make a significant improvement in the life of the patient. Like the other practitioners with whom I spoke, he also had a convincing observation of why his approach made an important contribution to health:

> In homeopathy, we do not depend on a disease classification as much as we do the symptoms present in the individual, their history, and their family history. This is because a single remedy may be able to cure very different diseases in different people. For instance, the homeopathic remedy Natrum muriaticum has been used with people who have had symptoms of allergies, vertigo, eczema, gall bladder problems (including acute gall bladder attacks), chronic constipation, grief-based depression, and multiple sclerosis. Given this unique capability of homeopathic remedies, you can see how it would be impossible to start from a general diagnosis and work one's way down to the specifics. This is not to say that in homeopathy we ignore physiology and pathology. We must know the difference between a simple barking cough and whooping cough, for instance, or between pneumonia and bronchitis. But,

again, it is the individual aspects of the case that will determine which remedy will cure.

Ultimately, it is the underlying predispositions, the inherited family patterns, which are resolved with the remedies. It is the underlying predisposition that is treated in order to resolve the symptoms. Homeopathy has addressed and cured people of many conditions for which conventional medicine has no solution, including psoriasis, eczema, multiple sclerosis, migraines, epilepsy, diverticulitis, depression, anxiety disorders, thyroid conditions, warts, cancer, and the list goes on. The reason the range of curability is so wide is because all homeopathy does, really, is remove the obstacles to the person's own vitality and that is what gets the person well. It isn't the remedy itself doing the healing; it just restores the body's natural vitality.

Mr. Wishart strongly affirmed the empirical basis of homeopathy and emphasized its repeatedly demonstrated therapeutic and curative properties. "So why aren't more people seeking homeopathic treatment?" He said that he gets that question often, and he replies to them:

> For those who scoff at homeopathy, there are 200 years of clinical data that support it. The oldest extant professional medical society in the United States is the American Institute of Homeopathy (the AMA was formed two years later). Homeopathy is widely accepted throughout Europe, India, and in Eastern European countries, as well as Mexico, Central, and South America. There is ample evidence for its efficacy.
>
> I am often asked, "Why, then if it works so well, don't more people do it?" I really don't know. I mention homeopathy often to friends who have health problems (and many times know the remedy that's needed) and some of them simply glaze-over. I guess it's not for them. I find this puz-

zling. As the question relates to physicians, I don't see why anyone whose mission it is to heal the sick would not at least be open-minded enough to investigate homeopathy.

These days, with a true crisis in healthcare, why would someone ignore homeopathy, acupuncture, and other well-documented, well-accepted medical systems? This is a question I suggest that every patient and physician ask themselves and then make a sincere effort to answer.

Alternatives for "Our Best Friends:" An Interview with Ronald Blaha, DC, CCSP, CAC

"Companion animals" seems too stoic a term for our household pets—members of the family for whom we have great fondness and attachment (sometimes more fondness than we have for blood relations). From the use of therapy dogs like Dr. Goldman's gentle Labrador, Booger, or therapy animals who visit long-term care facilities (what have more commonly been called "nursing homes"), companion animals are a balm for our emotional and physical well-being. We might not typically go for a walk in the neighborhood in freezing weather, but when our dog needs to "go outside" we comply to their physical needs. They keep us active and motivate us. They help us to age with good humor and patience. This is one reason that I got a dog before I had children. I needed to develop my patience!

When counseling with people who struggle with loneliness, there are times when I suggest their considering a companion animal. We need relationships and handle life's changes and stages better when we are less self-centered and consider the welfare of others, including the animal inhabitants with whom we share this planet.

When I saw the directory listing for animal chiropractic, I did a double-take. There is chiropractic medicine for animals?

Absolutely! For many professional animal handlers and breeders, animal chiropractic is not something to sneer at, but a vital approach to their animal's well-being. This section on complementary alternative medicine would not be complete without an alternative medical option for those members of our household that are our companions, friends, and a part of the family.

Dr. Ron Blaha is a Certified Animal Chiropractor in addition to his degree as a Doctor of Chiropractic Medicine, and certifications as a Chiropractic Sports Practitioner and Accupuncturist. His skills are sought throughout the North Texas area by animal lovers, dog breeders, horse enthusiasts, and greyhound racing organizations.

I came to the interview wondering: "What leads someone to seek Animal Chiropractic Certification, a field still rather new and only recently coming on the radar of the general public?" I knew Dr. Blaha as my chiropractor, and I knew of his passion for both chiropractic and holistic patient care, but I wanted to hear his thoughts that led to his present use of chiropractic in animal health care. As I expected, he convincingly laid out its benefits for animals and their owners, while commenting on the future of this unique field:

> I take a truly holistic approach to my patients' well-being and companion animals are essential for many people's emotional and physical well-being. Studies have shown that people who have companion animals such as dogs and cats have less stress and less depression. To keep their pets healthy, I wanted to offer chiropractic for them as well.
>
> I have worked with many greyhound owners because that breed is especially prone to spinal problems. There was a dog that could not get in or out of the vehicle without assistance. After one chiropractic treatment, he was jumping up into the car seat!

As people learn of these types of success stories, we will see wider acceptance and usage as they discover its benefits for their companion animals, horses, and other animals. We don't question the need for veterinary medicine, and with the proven effectiveness of chiropractic, animal chiropractic also makes sense as an essential component of animal health.

Alternatives to Prescription Drugs

Herbs, vitamins, dietary supplements, and homeopathic remedies are all alternatives to prescription drugs that many have found a godsend for their health. As is true with prescription medications, some treatments are more effective than others. One of the ironies that I have found in the "herbal-versus-prescription" battle is that some prescription medicines are also made from naturally occurring substances—penicillin and some cancer drugs come to mind. To simply claim that all herbal remedies are better because they are "natural" is tantamount to claiming that all surgery is unwarranted because surgery is not a naturally occurring phenomenon.

You have seen the advertisements on television and magazines and heard the claims touted by acclaimed radio personalities. We are told that there are great benefits to be had from these supplements that surpass many prescribed drugs. According to scientific research by respected pharmacologists, some of those claims are true.

Two of the most popular dietary supplements purchased by people middle-aged and over are glucosamine and chondroitin. These are used in the treatment of osteoarthritis, a painful inflammatory condition of the joints. *Geriatrics and Aging*, a clinical publication read by gerontologists and other medical professionals, published an article called, "Alternative Medicine that Actually Works?" The conclusion of the article, which specifically examined glucosamine and chondroitin in the treatment of osteoarthritis, was that these two over-the-counter supplements were "safe, superior to placebo, and as effective as non-steroidal anti-inflammatory drugs (NSAIDs) in relieving symptoms of osteoarthritis." Put one in the win column for alternative medicine.[60]

Still, not every alternative medication is as effective, and some can have some serious interactions with prescription drugs. Extreme caution should be used when combining dietary and herbal supplements with medication prescribed by physicians. Many pharmacists and some physicians have become more familiar with herbal and prescription pharmaceutical interaction now that herbal remedies are very commonly used, so consult professional advice before mixing the two.

According to another article in *Geriatrics and Aging*, here are some common herbal medicines and their potential interactions with drugs commonly prescribed for older people.

Table 4—Herbs and Possible Interactions[61]

Herb	Common Use	Drug	Possible Interactions (Reported in some patients)
Ginkgo Bilboa	Remedy for memory loss	Aspirin, Anticoagulants such as Heparin	Increased risk of bleeding. Long-term use has been linked to subdural hematomas (bleeding in the brain) and spontaneous hemorrhage.
Ginseng	Improve concentration	Digoxin (Cardiac drug), Warfarin (Anticoagulant), Phenelzine (Anti-depressant)	May elevate digoxin levels in blood. Diminishes effectiveness of Warfarin, increasing clotting risk. Serious manic side-effects when taken with Phenelzine.
Kava	Remedy for anxiety and insomnia	Alcohol, antidepressants, barbiturates, Levodopa (Parkinson's drug), benzodiazepines (sedatives)	May increase the drug's actions causing excessive hypnotic effect—particularly with alcohol. Alcohol significantly increases Kava's toxicity. Decreases the effectiveness of Levodopa in Parkinson's patients. May also have additive effects with anti-clotting drugs and certain types of antidepressants.
Valerian	Mild sedative for insomnia	Benzodiazepines (sedatives)	Potentiates their effects thus causing increased sedation and risk of falls, especially in older people.

St. John's Wort	Treatment for depression	Warfarin (Anticoagulant), Digoxin (Cardiac drug), Theophylline (Respiratory drug), Cyclosporine (immunosup-pressant), HIV medication, Antidepressants	Diminishes effectiveness of some drugs by interfering with how the body metabolizes them. Two cases of heart transplant rejection due to interaction with cyclosporine have been reported. May increase the potency of some anti-depressants causing greatly increased risk of side-effects including headache, gastrointestinal upset, restlessness, tremor, and changes in mental status.

Food Smarts

Good nutrition is crucial to good health. Exercise and good genes can only take us so far if we do not consider the impact that the food we eat has upon our bodies. The old adage, "An apple a day keeps the doctor away," is supported by scientific research about what makes a healthy diet. So, what are we supposed to eat to be healthy?

Generally, most physicians and nutritionists will tell you that a balanced diet is best. Again, each body is unique and your particular needs must consider your metabolism, physiology, medical history, and lifestyle. A 2,000-calorie diet might be only a fraction of the nutrition required by an athlete or teenager. Olympian Michael Phelps consumes 12,000 calories per day when in training![62]

In 2005, the United States Department of Agriculture (USDA) and Health and Human Services (HHS) co-published "Dietary Guidelines for Americans." This eighty-four-page document was first published in 1980 and is revised by these two agencies every five years. Concisely, it states that a balanced diet:

- Emphasizes fruits, vegetables, whole grains, and fat-free or low-fat milk and milk products
- Includes lean meats, poultry, fish, beans, eggs, and nuts; and
- Is low in saturated fats, *trans* fats, cholesterol, salt (sodium), and added sugars.[63]

The following information is based on United States Department of Agriculture and physician recommendations, but always consult your healthcare provider to learn what is best for your particular body's needs. Certainly, this is not an exhaustive list, either of all nutrients or of all food sources for the nutrients named. This is a good start to key nutritional needs and sources that contribute to a healthy and balanced diet.

Antioxidant/Folate-Rich Foods

Why you need it: Antioxidants fight-off "free radicals" that attack blood vessel walls and lead to atherosclerosis. There are indications that they can aid in the prevention of Alzheimer's Disease and other brain disorders.[64]

Where you get it: Any dark/bright-colored fruit or vegetable such as tomatoes, grapes, or apples (the "Delicious" variety has more nutrients in the skin than any other apple) and also leafy green vegetables. If diet is lacking, 400 mg. of folic acid as a supplement is a minimum recommended amount.[65]

Omega-3 Fatty Acids

Why you need it: Omega-3 fatty acids are recommended as a supplement that research suggests may slow the onset of Alzheimer's disease. Most physicians will tell you that a diet that includes fish and dietary fish oil supplements helps to lower triglycerides and reduces the risk of heart attack, cardiac arrhythmia, and stroke. Like antioxidants, omega-3 fatty acids can also slow down the process that causes hardening of the arteries and can help to lower blood pressure in patients with hypertension.

Where you get it: According to the Mayo Clinic website, "Dietary sources of omega-3 fatty acids include fish oil and certain plant/nut oils. Fish oil contains both docosahexaenoic acid (DHA) and eicosapentaenoic acid (EPA), while some nuts (English walnuts) and vegetable oils (canola, soybean, flaxseed/linseed, and olive) contain alpha-linolenic acid (ALA)." [66]

Various articles in recent news and health publications warn that if you are taking fish-oil supplements, check the label for purity to avoid lead, heavy metals, or other contaminants sometimes found in fish and fish byproducts.

Cholesterol-Lowering Food

Why you need it: The lower your LDL (bad cholesterol), the better your cardiovascular health—the pipes tend not to get clogged. The higher your HDL (good cholesterol), the result is the same.

Where you get it: Oatmeal and oat-based cereal. Also, avoid fatty foods–saturated fats in particular, and all trans-fats. (See below)

High-Fiber Foods

Why you need it: Fiber is essential for colon health. The small intestine is where most nutrients are absorbed that fuel your body. The large intestine (colon) is where water is absorbed. Keep it working well and you will maintain your overall nutrition and feel great while avoiding constipation.

Where you get it: Wheat, oats, whole grains, bran, soy, baked beans, almonds, pistachios, bananas, apples, pears, berries, and melons such as cantaloupe.

Low-Fat Foods

Why you need it: Low-fat food means heart-healthy food that does not clog vital arteries and helps avoid strokes.

Where you get it: Read dietary information labels on the food that you purchase to avoid foods high in saturated and trans fats. Here is an important tip: Current labeling laws do not require nutrition labeling on food prepared in-store, such as many of the baked goods you buy at your local grocery. I am fond of the cinnamon coffee-cake on sale each week at my local *Kroger* grocery store. Since it is made at the store's bakery, there is no detailed information about fat content, but the *ingredients* are required to be listed on the label. When you see partially hydrogenated oils, take note! That is the source of trans fat or trans fatty acids. Trans fat is a man-made byproduct of hydrogenation, a process that increases the shelf-life of oil used in baking. Without it we wouldn't have such things as "Crisco" brand shortening or margarine. Trans fat lowers HDL cholesterol levels in your blood (the kind you want) and raises LDL cholesterol levels (which is not what you want). I encourage you to do some web-surfing for an explanation and history of trans-fatty acids. It is eye-opening.

Low-fat dairy products such as skim milk are one example of nutritional and low-fat foods. Again, read the nutrition information label to avoid assumptions. Two percent milk has only a fraction less fat than whole milk, so unless you are feeding a child or someone whose diet requires whole milk, skim is best. Low-fat or non-fat yogurt is another good choice in the dairy case. Both can be a good source of calcium and vitamin D, as many are enriched with these.

High Protein Foods

Why you need it: Protein is an essential part of any diet and contributes to health on the cellular level as well as muscle development. Protein is one of the primary components of our body, needed for bones, teeth, skin, nerves, blood components, and anti-bodies. Too much protein is stored as fat and tasks the liver and kidneys.[67]

Where you get it: Lean meats, beans and legumes, dairy foods, soy, and protein supplements.

Nutritional Supplements

Though this is not an exhaustive list, as that would be unwieldy given the nature of this book, these are some of the most common products marketed as dietary/nutritional supplements:

- Multi-vitamin/mineral
- Vitamin B complex
- Vitamins C, D, and E
- Beta-carotene

- Omega-3 fatty acids
- Folic acid
- Zinc
- Iron
- Acidophilus
- Black cohosh
- Evening primrose oil
- Echinacea
- Fiber
- Garlic
- Ginkgo bilboa
- Fish oil
- Glucosamine and/or chondroitin sulfate
- St. John's wort
- Saw palmetto. [68]

Remember this important tip when choosing vitamins and nutritional supplements: supplements that have the USP (United States Pharmacoepia) rating on the label for purity and absorption are best. You are assured that you are getting the dosage printed on the label. Unless it says "USP" or "Assured Release," your body may not actually be getting what the label claims. As with any medication or supplement, over-the-counter or otherwise, discuss your particular health needs with your physician or health-care provider. Not everyone needs supplements and your unique health concerns may make supplements unwise for you. Pharmacists and nutritionists can also be a good source for advice as you develop a plan of good nutritional health. As noted in his interview, Dr.

Horoda highly recommends a blood test to determine your levels of these most significant vitamin/mineral/and supplemental needs. Here is some helpful information on the most commonly used of these.

Calcium

You lose calcium daily. If you don't replace it, the body draws it from the bones, making you more susceptible to fractures and some ligament injuries. Calcium-fortified orange juice, milk, and dairy products are good sources. Antacid tablets can have dual benefit as a good source of calcium and an aid in treating acid reflux disease or simple indigestion. Taking Vitamin D with calcium aids in its absorption, which is why some calcium supplements include the vitamin as a part of the supplement.

Daily Multiple Vitamin

Why do you need to take a multi-vitamin daily? Because nobody's diet is perfect. Almost everyone, including children, can benefit from a daily multi-vitamin. Check with your pediatrician before adding this to your child's diet. Discuss with your physician if you have any medical conditions, such as kidney or liver disease, which may exclude you from this standard recommendation by the American Medical Association and the Center for Disease Prevention.

Save your money and buy a quality store brand rather than a name brand. Look for the USP rating on the label for purity and potency. Compare labels. A store-brand at my local grocer of a USP-rated daily multi-vitamin contained exactly the same vitamin supplements as the nationally advertised name brand and was almost three-dollars less for the same quantity.

Iron

Iron supplements are beneficial for most women and for some children, but are no longer recommended for men over forty unless advised by a physician. Iron is believed to increase the risk of clotting in men, which can lead to stroke or heart attack. Iron aids women in staving-off anemia which can be influenced by menstruation and poor diet.

Antioxidant Supplements

There are many different supplements that provide antioxidant properties. One simple way of approaching this is to think ACE. Vitamins A, C, and E are primary antioxidants that improve vascular health, strengthen the immune system, and generally contribute to your overall health. There are varying opinions about what doses of these you should take. As with many vitamin supplements, extremely high doses can cause significant side-effects and even liver damage. High doses of vitamin A, particularly the non-water-soluble type, can result in nausea and even contribute to hair loss (don't worry guys, that is only in really large daily doses). Too much vitamin E, when taken with aspirin or NSAID's, such as ibuprofen, can lower your clotting factor to the point that it increases your risk of bleeding. Recent studies have questioned if vitamin E increases the risk of vascular disease, particularly strokes, but it is still used and recommended in many cases. [69]

Bottom-line, you need all three, but they are best gotten through eating a balanced diet. At the very least, take your multi-vitamin. If your multi-vitamin doesn't provide the recommended minimum daily requirement (RDA) of A, C, and E, and neither does your diet, then take a supplement. I take twice the RDA of vitamins A and C, and let my multi-vitamin provide me with the vitamin E that I do not get from foods. A daily baby-aspirin can have as much vascular benefit as vitamin E, with other plusses as well. Patients with stomach or Glycemic Index problems, or who are allergic, may need to forego the aspirin. Check with your pharmacist, nutritionist, or health-care provider for the latest news on antioxidants because findings of new studies are frequently being released.

Other Mineral Supplements

I have already covered calcium and iron. Because we are each unique "chemistry sets" or bio-chemical organisms, the needs of each individual may vary. Taking too much of some supplements can cause hypersensitivity to taste and smell, gastrointestinal upset, and, in some cases, hypersensitivity to ultraviolet light. I have personally experienced the hypersensitive smell, so I cut back on minerals and use a daily multivitamin without the mineral supplement. As I mentioned above, studies suggest that men not take iron supplements unless recommended by their physician, so that is another reason for guys to choose a vitamin sans the minerals.

Some acne patients have reported that additional zinc can be beneficial, as have patients who are in the initial stages of a cold virus, cold sore, or herpes-simplex mouth ulcer. Some of the leading cold-relief medications are primarily made of zinc (e.g. Zicam™, Cold-eeze®).

Chromium has been shown to aid in the metabolism of sugar. With the growing trend in obesity and diabetes, some in the medical community recommend including chromium supplements as a part of weight-loss program.

Selenium combines with proteins to create antioxidants that slow cellular damage. It aids the immune system and the regulation of thyroid function.

There is no one right answer for all circumstances, so take the time and effort to ask a nutritionist in your community (consider consulting the dietician of a local hospital) or speak with a pharmacist. This could be a part of your self-care plan to have a scheduled consultation with a nutritional expert and determine what is right for you.

Avoid pseudo-nutritionists at your local health club who may only be trying to sell you the club's protein and whey supplements. It is worth paying a fee to consult with a professional who can give you a long-term plan than to get a "free" consultation with someone whose goal is to sell you expensive dietary supplements. Above all, keep a common sense approach, and do not be afraid to ask questions of more than one healthcare provider if you question the advice you receive.

For Reflection

1. What changes would be helpful for you to make in order for you to physically feel better and healthier?

2. Do you think that any cultural attitudes we have contribute to over-eating and our general habit as a nation of being over-consumers? Consider our attitude toward the consumption of fossil fuels. It took the 2008 economic crisis and historic high oil prices to increase the use of mass transit and the demand of fuel-efficient vehicles in the United States. Other industrialized nations with healthy economies have successfully incorporated the wide use of mass transit into their national consciousness

for years. Why do you think Americans have been so resistant to such change?

3. How does our attitude toward life and health impact the well-being of poor and impoverished families in third-world countries? By our consumption and spending, how is our stewardship affecting their lives? Do you believe that hunger and poverty could be reduced by a significant change in the behavior of consumers? What would it take for that to happen?

TAKING AN ALTERNATE ROUTE

Rethinking Stereotypes of Aging, Relationships, and Retirement

"It's time we stopped dismissing middle age as the beginning of the end. Research suggests that at forty, the brain's best years are still ahead."

—Gene Cohen, M.D., Ph.D.[70]

"I shall die young, at whatever age the experience occurs."

—Ruth Bernhard
101-year-old internationally acclaimed photographer

"Your food stamps will be stopped effective March 1992 because we received notice that you passed away. May God bless you. You may reapply if there is a change in your circumstances."

—Letter to a family
from the Department of Social Services,
Greenville, South Carolina[71]

Stereotypes, Fear, and Prejudice

Cultures reflect their stereotypes, fear, and prejudice in their behavior and choices. As a society, our perspective of aging and any fear or stereotypes we associate with growing old are seen in how we provide for older adults, including social customs and legislative policies. Dr. Tom Kirkwood, with a strong and compelling voice, speaks to all of us about our disrespect of an aging population:

> There is an unfortunate tendency to see the graying of the world's population as a disaster in the making instead of the twofold triumph that it really is. Firstly, we have managed—not a moment too soon—to begin to bring soaring population growth under control. Secondly, we have succeeded, through vaccination, antibiotics, sanitation, nutrition, education, and so on, in bringing death rates down. If it turns out now that we lack the will and strategies to accommodate the elderly people that result from these successes, and to realize their potential as a benefit not a burden, then perhaps we should seriously question whether as a species, we can justly continue to conduct our affairs under the grandiose title of *Homo sapiens.*"[72]

Imagine your life is an hour-glass, with sand emptying from the upper chamber to fill the lower chamber. What is your perspective? You can choose to keep your eye on the upper chamber and worry about how much sand is left or you can discover that it is more fun to watch the sand in the lower chamber and see what shape it takes.

We choose our perspective and our attitude. We choose whether or not to allow our worry and fear to consume us. We choose optimism or skepticism. We choose to be frustrated or to allow the unstoppable current to carry us to new opportunities, even if we would rather be upstream than downstream. If we cannot change the current, we can choose to find opportunity from the direction that it takes us. As challenging as this can be, we take encouragement and inspiration from those around us who create opportunities even when the current of life seems to be against them.

Our culture, like many others, admires persons who achieve personal success and make remarkable accomplishments in a positive way. Persons such as Oprah Winfrey, Michael Jordan, Jimmy Carter, Cesar Chavez, Barack Obama, Neil Armstrong, Lady Bird Johnson, Billy Graham, Nelson Mandela, Walter Cronkite, Sandra Day O'Connor, Colin Powell, Gerald Ford, Nolan Ryan, Thurgood Marshall, Mother Teresa, Ellen Ochoa, Pope John Paul II, Muhammad, Hillary Clinton, Michelle Wie, Mohandas Gandhi, Ben Nighthorse Campbell, Dwayne Johnson, Martin Luther King, Jr., Coretta Scott King, and Rosa Parks bear witness to personal accomplishment and overcoming obstacles. These, along with many other everyday, unsung heroes who work hard, make wise choices, demonstrate good stewardship, share their gifts and work to serve others, are an inspiration to us all. We need such role-models, for as longevity increases, quality of life is even more essential for all of our days, not just the young and mid-years of life.

People are living longer. We have made great advances in cardiac care. New medications, such as "clot-buster" drugs, can be used to stop heart attacks and strokes at time of onset. There are greater numbers of well-trained first responders than ever before due to advances in EMS delivery. Life-saving cardiac defibrillators have been made automatic and placed in many community buildings for use by the general public. There are now treatments for historically impossible-to-treat malignancies such as pancreatic and lung cancer.

We are more informed about our health and our bodies than at any time in history. We are more aware of the role of exercise, nutrition, and dietary supplements for better health and longevity. We have new pharmaceuticals that offer amazing results in lowering cholesterol, stabilizing blood pressure, and warding off the complications of diabetes.

As medical science gains knowledge of disease processes, we are better able to diagnose maladies and prescribe treatment. Decades ago, there were occasions when someone's cause of death was listed in generic ways such as "heart attack" or "old age." I saw one death certificate where the cause of death was listed as "not listening to her doctor!" We now know that there were actually other disease processes—then unidentified—that were involved. We not only view death and disease differently, we are also beginning to view the stages of life differently.

According to aging trends author, Maddy Dychtwald, retiring baby boomers do not consider themselves over the hill, and they have redefined the word "young." She writes:

> 'Young' is no longer defined by a specific age, but by a life of energy and vitality. The new definition of retirement is to engage, to reinvent, and to seek freedom. It is no longer a linear life movement from birth, to education, to marriage or work, to retiring, and finally death, but a full 'cyclic' life progression of 'ageless aging,'[73]

A Fresh Perspective on Relationships: A Community of Care

The biblical book of The Acts of the Apostles shares a snapshot of the early church living together as a sharing community of care:

Awe came upon everyone, because many wonders and signs were being done by the apostles. All who believed were together and had all things in common; they would sell their possessions and goods and distribute the proceeds to all, as any had need. Day be day, as they spent much time together in the temple, they broke bread at home and ate their food with glad and generous hearts, praising God and having the goodwill of all the people. And day by day, the Lord added to their number those who were being saved.

Acts 2:43—47

This is a great lesson in how community is meant to be. I am not speaking of politics or socialism, but a reconsideration of how we view relationships. A community of care is where the needs of others are foremost on the minds of the whole.

One of the most basic characteristics of this model of community, which may be overlooked in its importance, is that they shared their meals in common—they ate together. There is something enormously satisfying in breaking the bread of life with those you love. There is satisfaction in sharing a meal with others because loneliness is replaced with companionship. There is camaraderie and even a sense of intimacy in eating together with another human being.

People gathered around a table while taking nourishment is a satisfying human experience that transcends race, culture, gender, or age and provides common ground that unites people and nourishes more than just our bodies. Bodies, minds, and souls are fed through the sustenance of shared fellowship. Loneliness is abated. Loneliness can be a crucial issue and becomes an even greater concern as our life circumstances change; spouses, partners, and/or friends die, and children grow up to move on with their own lives.

Another basic characteristic of true community reflected in this passage is the sharing of possessions and resources. There is no need. There is no want. There is no one left out. There is no one alone. There is no one who is not welcome at the table. There is always room for one more. For me, this is the image of what the New Testament calls "the kingdom of God!" This is the essence of the wholeness described by the Hebrew word, *shalom*, when applied to the human family.

We do not often come very close to this image of true community. We may share resources freely through monetary gifts to United Way, the Red Cross, or some other helping agency in order to help those in need around us. We may share resources grudgingly through taxes that support government-sponsored programs for children, senior adults, and the impoverished. We may donate clothing that we do not want, belongings that we no longer need, or things that we perceive as garbage in order to have a tax deduction, yet do it in the guise of aiding the lives of those on the street. This may be as close as we get to "having all things in common;" it is not very close.

For life to be rich, full, and peaceful both now and through-out our days of growing older, it is vital that we discover the true importance of giving ourselves away. When the tsunamis, hurricanes, and earthquakes of 2005 and 2008 occurred, people responded to the undeniable human need. There was an international outpouring of help through cash contributions and material goods. The devastation was so extensive and the images via twenty-first century news-gathering so compelling, that people responded from around the world. People respond when the need is genuine, the cause is just, and the reality is perceived.

Caring community is not unlike the biblical descriptions of the kingdom of heaven. As such, it is also not some abstract place "up above" where "heavenly hosts" hang out. Caring community is whenever and wherever two or more people come together and think of each other without merely thinking of only themselves.

In foxholes and fancy sanctuaries, nursing homes and neighborhoods, mansions and modest apartments, caring community can be in our midst. After all, if we say that heaven means so much to us, then let us live today as we say we will live then. If caring community is so important, then let us make it a central part of our lives and band together with people who share the vision of love, justice, and service. When we do, amazing things begin to happen!

Caring Community in Action

Early one Tuesday morning, a young Hispanic man knocked on the locked glass doors of a church where I served as the senior pastor. Mary Bassett, a retired teacher and senior adult member of the congregation, happened to be inside. She was preparing for a women's meeting, but she stopped what she was doing and went to the door to talk with the man. Being alone, she did not wish to let him in, so Mary asked what he needed. She discerned that he was in spiritual and emotional pain and in need of the pastor. She summoned me to the church and I learned that I needed a translator to speak to him. Kurt Kauffman, a bi-lingual parishioner, left work to provide translation for us and we sat with the young man as he poured out the pain of his story.

Being from another country, he did not know anyone here except some immoral co-workers who had been a very bad influence upon him. His mother had told him that whenever he needed help, he should go to a church; so he stopped when he saw the cross on our building. Problems are not resolved overnight, but as the weeks unfolded, his story began to take a very positive turn. We connected the man to a Spanish-speaking church near where he lived. He had never before been committed to any faith, but he began attending services that week, and soon asked to be baptized. Not long afterward, he chose to dedicate his life in Christian service and entered seminary in his home country. He is excited about what God has done and is doing in his life.

This is a remarkable story in very many ways. So many things could have stood in the way of this young man's redemption from his desperate circumstances. A senior adult could have chosen not to be bothered by a persistent visitor knocking on the door before office hours. I could have told him to come back another time when it was more convenient. The translator could have said that he was too busy at work. The pastor to whom we referred him could have chosen not to devote the time required at this critical point of his spiritual journey. Because people chose to respond in kind—to respond with the same grace and faith that God gives each one of us—a life was touched and changed.

The heart of the Church of Jesus Christ is not rules, but relationships. Sharing love and joy is so much more important than being sanctimonious and self-righteous. All who identify themselves as a part of the body of Christ hold an important role, for each are called to be a witness to and example of unconditional love. A community of care is rooted in such loving actions and attitudes that transform the world one life at a time. Christians may do it because they desire to be Christlike, but whatever one's faith or motivation, offering care to others is the essence of what is most noble about humanity— the capacity to grow beyond self and to reach out to connect with God and each other.

Being the Best You Can Be

In my mind, I can still hear the hypnotic and gentle sound of a man's voice melodiously reading from a western novel. The sound came from the electronic speaker of my father's "Talking Book" player provided by the Lighthouse for the Blind. It is how he read—listening to the voice of another transforming the printed word into an enunciated recorded message of prose. My father, blinded by an explosion at age twenty-eight, loved Westerns, biographies, and non-fiction. National Geographic and Newsweek were his favorite magazines. He couldn't visually read them, but he read by listening to them.

I tried purchasing novels in audio form for my Dad, which he politely accepted, but it wasn't his interest. He was on a first-name basis with his librarian at the Texas State Library for the Blind, and she kept him supplied via parcel post with recordings of his favorite reading material. Initially, they were distributed on vinyl phonographic records and then the media progressed to cassette tapes.

Dad was being the best that he could be and that was his outlook for which he can always be remembered and commended. Some would look on him with pity or sympathy, or think of him as not being especially significant. Quite to the contrary, I looked at him and saw a hero. He was a strong man of character who overcame enormous challenges, primarily the industrial explosion that cost him his sight. At the time of the accident, he was engaged to be married to the woman who would become the mother of my sister and me. By entering into marriage with him, mother also became an example of perseverance—a heroine whose devotion to her husband and children would dominate her entire life's journey.

Dad has demonstrated for others the importance of self-sufficiency, education, and honesty. He lived out the values of love of family and love of God. His sense of humor was delightful, and his ability to make something creative and utilitarian out of spare parts and leftover junk was utterly amazing. He ingeniously created a helpful and practical tool from a piece of aluminum siding, a part of a metal storm door, a strip of rubber from a garden hose, and a broom handle to pull my recycling bin to the curb without straining my back!

Someone wrote to me once on the occasion of the death of a member of my congregation. They said that we all know people who we think of as worse than us or better than us, but the true test of human fulfillment is someone who is being the best that they can be. Dad was simply being the best that he could be. Dad lived in the moment while neither ignoring the future nor failing to learn from the past. Rare people live this truth and model it for others. Nature also teaches us this lesson when we pause to notice.

Living in the Now

As I am writing this chapter, I am on Whidbey Island sitting on the porch of a rented bungalow in the small village of Langley, Washington. There is a small cotton-tail rabbit that is playing amidst the wildflowers and shrubbery. Two other rabbits have now joined him in frolic, and their scurrying means that all four of us are having fun. To my amazement, he approaches quite casually, coming within three feet of my chair before hopping off the other way. He, like most animals—except for the majority of humankind—lives in the moment. He is being the best rabbit that he can be. He follows his instincts, which guide him to fulfill his basic needs of food, water, procreation, and survival.

This brings him enjoyment. He is content. He neither fears the future nor the aging that is to come in his short lifespan.

Humanity may have intellect that leads us to think and envision beyond the present, but that same intellect can overlook the present and allow us to miss the precious moment that is now. Our present matters as much as our future. Reality is often what we make it to be and our reality can be filled with delight or with dread.

Growing older is a normal and significant part of this journey called life. Life's journey is filled with wondrous variations, surprising turns, challenging obstacles, steep inclines, and thrilling downhill runs. Whether going down or up, the ride is still important. Goals give us something for which to strive and serve to keep us focused, but the route we take toward fulfilling our goals is just as important as accomplishing them. If our destination is solely our focus, we will have missed the journey—and the journey is the ride of our life!

The Waste of "What Might Have Been"

Yesterdays can hold many fond memories, great achievements, and celebrated successes. Our past history can also be a source of burden and regret when we choose to stay there and not move on.

For several years, I regularly videotaped a favorite television series—even if I was watching it live. If, during the program, I had rewound the tape to review a previous scene, I would have missed the live action as well as the opportunity of taping it. Apparently, others have had this problem, as TiVo® and digital video recorders (DVRs) were invented to resolve this troubling dilemma. Thanks to these electronic marvels, you can stop or rewind live TV programs without missing any portion of the broadcast. Unfortunately, real life has no TiVo®. Moments missed when we focus on the past instead of the present are moments lost forever. [74]

How much time we waste on worry and what might have been! The long list of "if only" carries with it a burden much heavier than the small phrase suggests:

- If only I had chosen a different career!
- If only I had said yes to that opportunity!
- If only I had made better choices!
- If only my parents had raised me differently!
- If only I had raised my children differently!
- If only I had come from a "better" family!
- If only I had married a different person!
- If only I had gotten a better education!
- If only I had worked harder!
- If only I had worked less and enjoyed life more!
- If only I had spent more time with my family!
- If only I had more money!
- If only I had more time!
- If only I had better health!
- If only I had fewer hardships!
- If only I had been dealt a better hand!
- If only I had done a better job with the hand I was dealt!
- If only I had it all to do over again!
- If only....

Hear and claim this truth:

Dwelling on yesterday's failures is perpetuating failure by wasting today and tomorrow.

By living in and focusing on the present, while refusing to rehearse past mistakes, disappointments, heartaches, failures, or tragedies, we:

- Gain time to enjoy today!
- Open possibilities for tomorrow!
- Allow time for creativity!
- Begin to heal from yesterday's hurts!
- Move from lingering over the past to learning from the past!
- Move from negativity ("I'll probably make the same dumb mistake again!") to possibility ("How can I reinvent my future by learning from my past?")
- Become the authentic, whole, and growing person whom God intends us to be!

God doesn't want us to live as broken people. God wants us to live as joyful people. God doesn't want us to stay as we are. God wants us to grow into what we can become. God doesn't want us to see life as a struggle with difficulties. God wants us to see life as a journey of opportunities.

Life can be tragic. "Crack babies" and "AIDS babies" begin life with bleak beginnings, but that need not be where they remain. One in seven children living in sub-Saharan Africa dies before the age of five, primarily due to malaria, malnutrition, or AIDS.[75] This tragic statistic must be and will be improved. *Sports Illustrated*, the United Methodist Church, NBA Cares, and the United Nations Foundation have partnered with other organizations to form the Nothing-but-Nets Campaign. The goal is to provide insecticide-treated mosquito netting to every person in every community and nation needing them in order to halt the epidemic of malaria that plagues the African continent.[76] The tragedies of life that we can work together to reverse make possible a world that is truly a community of caring. We can waste time with "what might have been" or work together toward what is good and just and possible.

When Dave Roever was severely burned by a phosphorous grenade in Viet Nam, he could have given up on life. He was badly disfigured, in a great deal of pain, and faced a formidable recovery. Dave chose to continue his journey by using the strength that he received from his faith in God. Because he chose to become more than he was and he refused to be stopped by the limitations life gave him, he has inspired and encouraged countless people to live lives of faith, hope, and possibility.[77]

If you waste your life by dwelling on what might have been—if you revisit yesterday's regrets long after the failures have passed—you are robbing yourself of the unexpected joy and possibilities that today can hold. If you medicate the memories of the past such that addictions to medication, illegal drugs, alcohol, food, sex, gambling, shopping, or spending develop, you will also miss the gift of living in the present. You can let go, with the help of God and the support of a caring network comprised of support groups (twelve-step groups if addiction is robbing you of living today), friends, family, mental health professionals, and spiritual friends/mentors. Make the effort. Take the steps. Live the life that today can hold for you by releasing the pain of yesterday.

Taking Stress Seriously

Stress is like poverty, people often think that there is nothing you can do about either one, so they do not try. Both are a curse to life and how we respond determines how they affect us and others.

For decades, I have acted like there is nothing I could do about stress and my career. That is not true. I can change my attitude toward stressors: tasks, people, or events. I can change my schedule to make more time for exercise and hobbies, even if it means going to bed or getting up earlier. I can reprioritize to avoid wasting time on the unimportant and having more time for the things I enjoy. I can seek others to hold me accountable to lifestyle changes. I can celebrate when I successfully reduce my stress and forgive myself when setbacks happen to my plan. After all, we all need plenty of "second chances."

Stress is a physiological reality that impacts our health just as surely as poor nutrition can affect us. Both of these impact our well-being. A University of California at Los Angeles (UCLA) study suggests that stress is not only physiological, but that the physiology of stress is different for men than it is for women:

> Scientists now suspect that hanging out with our friends can actually counteract the kind of stomach-quivering stress most of us experience on a daily basis. A landmark UCLA study suggests that women respond to stress with a cascade of brain chemicals that cause us to make and maintain friendships with other women. It's a stunning find that has turned five decades of stress research—most of it on men—upside down.

"Until this study was published, scientists generally believed that when people experience stress, they trigger a hormonal cascade that revs the body to either stand and fight or flee as fast as possible," explains Laura Cousin Klein, Ph.D., now an Assistant Professor of Biobehavioral Health at Penn State University and one of the study's authors. It's an ancient survival mechanism left over from the time we were chased across the planet by saber-toothed tigers.

Now the researchers suspect that women have a larger behavioral repertoire than just fight or flight. In fact, says Dr. Klein, it seems that when the hormone oxytocin is released as part of the stress responses in a woman, it buffers the fight or flight response and encourages her to tend children and gather with other women instead. When she actually engages in this tending or befriending, studies suggest that more oxytocin is released, which further counters stress and produces a calming effect. This calming response does not occur in men, says Dr. Klein, because testosterone—which men produce in high levels when they're under stress—seems to reduce the effects of oxytocin. Estrogen; she adds, seems to enhance it.[78]

This study is fascinating and points to the significant biochemical differences associated with gender. It may add further insight into women's longevity over men. If women are biologically more social, it would also help to explain their tendency to have lower blood pressure and cholesterol than many men. Social ties reduce stress and stress-related diseases including cardiovascular disease. As Dr. Klein puts it, "There's no doubt that friends are helping us live longer."[79]

A Piece of Wisdom That Can Change Your Life Forever

Wisdom and knowledge are different. You may have the knowledge of how to build a lawn mower, but to wisely entice a young person to use it on your lawn without financial compensation—that is wisdom! Wisdom transcends knowledge and overwhelms ignorance.

Wisdom clears away life's dense jungle of gibberish and obfuscation. Wisdom breaks through destructive rhetoric and angst to silence the loudmouth and vanquish the wicked. Wisdom cuts to the heart or stirs the heart to quicken. Wisdom, in its season, yields both peace and anguish. Wisdom knows when to "be still and know," and when to cry out above the silence of apathy.

Wisdom knows this truth that is one of the most important lessons of life:

> *Stop worrying about what others think of you and listen to your heart.*

God is there in your heart. God is in the still, small voice that longs to be heard. God is in the sound that has been squelched. God is in the life deprived of liberty that longs to be set free. God is in the talent that has been hidden because of those around that fail to comprehend or embrace genius.

In the biblical book of 1 Kings, chapter seventeen, the story is told of the prophet, Elijah, and a widow whom he encountered. Elijah and the widow, with the help of God, supported each other during a three-year drought. The story also demonstrates that a drought—substitute the term "tough times"—need not be only bad, but can be a time of good.

Our society tends to think of God as one to blame in the face of natural disasters—the catastrophic hurricanes on the southern coast of the United States, the terrifying tsunamis of Indonesia, and the devastating earthquakes in Pakistan, China, Kashmir, and Haiti. Drought times can be an opportunity to discover God at work for good, because (for a change) we are looking for God to be about the task of blessing and creating hope. We can see the signs of hope that God has wrought, when we are willing to look through eyes of faith. It is a redemptive quality of such disastrous times that through terrible trials in dire circumstances we can, upon reflection when calm has finally come, find ourselves more keenly aware of God's presence and may find ourselves even stronger because of it.

Drought times can be an opportunity to learn something from our difficulty or through our experience of disquiet and discomfort. We can choose to examine how we handle aging, suffering, resentment, grief, failure, disappointment, despair, isolation, or waiting. Drought times can be an opportunity to re-examine how we handle relationships and how we look at other people. What might we learn about ourselves from even the difficult people whom we encounter? Do we own our poor choices, negative traits, destructive habits, or self-centeredness that contribute to failed marriages or damaged friendships?

May we grow closer to God in good times as well as the bad and discover that God's presence along our journey can make any time a good time to be both hopeful and alive. It is a blessing for me to share the journey with you.

For Reflection

1. What is one thing that you have yet to do to "live to be your own best self?"

2. What is your time and life waster? Is it an "If only..." "What

might have been…" or "I failed to…" What is your next step toward letting that go?

3. How do you and/or the organization, church, synagogue, or mosque to which you belong fulfill your calling to be a community of caring? What is it that you can still do or what opportunity are you ignoring? What is holding you back?

TORCH BEARERS
People Who Light the Way

"Just as when weaving one reaches the end with fine threads woven throughout, so is the life of humans."

—Buddha

"In my beginning is my end...In my end is my beginning."

—T.S. Eliot, "East Coker"

"If you have gathered nothing in your youth, how can you find anything in your old age?"

—Ecclesiasticus 25:3 (The Jerusalem Bible)

Ordinary People—Extraordinary Examples

Torch bearers—we all know some of them. They are extraordinary leaders, everyday homemakers, peace-making soldiers, remarkable athletes, living examples and ordinary people. They are people of conviction and compassion, discipline and daring, with faith in the future and encouragement for those around them. Life is not easy. It takes courage, stamina, and perseverance to continue the journey. Such is the example of men and women who live large by living with confidence rather than fear.

Every human being has fears, whether healthy fear or otherwise. No one escapes this world without encountering obstacles that may make us tremble or leave us doubting ourselves. The distinction of persons whom I call torch bearers of life is that they are willing to face life's uncertainties, terrors, and troubles and live boldly with conviction, faith, and passion. Above all, torch bearers are people of passion. They are passionate about what they believe; their passion defines what they are willing to live for or die for. Sometimes, their courage and contributions are not appreciated until they are gone.

A mother or father, sister or brother, friend or co-worker, spouse or companion can be a torch-bearer. Perhaps our relationship with them was not that good, or perhaps we simply took them for granted. We may have had expectations of them that they never fulfilled. A parent often fails to live up to our fullest expectations, and then we appreciate the difficulty of the task when we become a parent ourselves. Bosses, teachers, coaches, ministers, professors, physicians, politicians, and other leaders whom we look up to are all broken people who do not always "get it right."

Sacrifices made by them may never be appreciated until long after they are gone. Sometimes, when we struggle with life ourselves, we realize that they were doing the very best they could. We may realize how high we set the bar for them, how little we understood them, or how unfairly we judged them. Perhaps we later come to understand that they were actually heroic in how they pressed on through difficulties which we ourselves could not have navigated.

Not Afraid to Lead: Willa Player, Ph.D.

Willa Player, Ph.D., lived to be ninety-four years of age. Her body died August 27, 2003, but her spirit and legacy continue to shine. Dr. Player was the first African-American woman to head a four-year college in the United States. She served as president of Bennett College in Greensboro, North Carolina, from 1955–1966, and had been a member of the faculty of that liberal arts college for women for twenty-four years prior to that. She hosted civil rights leader, the Reverend Dr. Martin Luther King, Jr., when other colleges and churches in Greensboro closed their doors to his message. Dr. Player stood up for students who were jailed for efforts to integrate restaurants, theaters, and other institutions. She faced intimidation by cruel bullies, threats of violence against herself and the institution that she served, times of financial uncertainty and economic drought, oppression, subjugation, and prejudice. Dr. Player rose up and stood firm when the torrent of injustice tried to wash away what she believed in. [80]

Some people are so busy worrying about dying that they are afraid of living. Dr. Player was not such a person. Torch bearers live with hope and with the conviction that no trepidation, devastation, or isolation is ever so deep as to be outside of hope's embrace.

Torch bearers are not perfect people. Like all of us, they are flawed and with their own fears, failures, and insecurities. Above all, they are hopeful people. They are loving, faithful, and persevering people.

West Texas Ranching Woman: Lilly Bell Kindley

Lilly Bell Kindley, my grandmother, was a wife, mother, and rancher. When my grandfather developed crippling rheumatoid arthritis and became bed-ridden, she assumed full responsibility for running a 737-acre ranch. During one of the worst droughts in Texas history, hay and feed were scarce. The federal government distributed certificates to ranch owners who were eligible to receive cattle feed through a United States Department of Agriculture program. Grandma Kindley took her paperwork and drove her pick-up truck to the train station in Graham, Texas, to collect the feed that was due to her.

Upon arriving at the station, she found work-hands from another large ranch loading all of the feed onto their trucks. She approached them and declared, "Some of that feed is mine!" They ignored her. She presented her certificates and told them that some of that feed belonged to her. The ranch hands still ignored her. She was emphatic and said, "This paperwork says that some of that feed is mine!"

"No ma'am," the lead worker responded, "this all belongs to our boss."

Going back to her truck, she reached behind the seat and pulled out a Winchester rifle that she kept there. It was meant to use on varmints such as rattlesnakes or coyotes, should she ever come upon one. Returning with the Winchester in hand, she said quite calmly, "This Winchester says that some of that feed is mine." The lead worker looked up at the now more-imposing, no-nonsense ranch owner and simply said, "Yes ma'am, where would you like us to put your feed?"

Life is not easy and its twists and turns can make for a rough ride. Perseverance and courage in the face of hardship and conflict testify to character and conviction. History has its characters, and their story can leave a legacy of inspiration and humor long after they have "ridden off into the sunset."

Professor, Counselor, Mentor, and Golfer: Charles F. Kemp, Ph.D.

Charles F. Kemp, Ph.D., was professor emeritus of Pastoral Care and Counseling at Texas Christian University in Fort Worth, Texas. He established the Pastoral Care and Counseling Center on the TCU campus, a facility which provided free or low-cost mental health services for all ages while training pastoral counselors. This alone would be a great legacy for anyone, but there was more to Dr. Kemp: he had an ardent passion for golf.

He worked with professional golfers, men and women of the PGA and LPGA, practicing sports psychology to help them through slumps in their careers. He wrote numerous books; some about counseling, some about the Bible, and some were about golf. For recreation, he traveled and played the best courses in the world. Following his retirement, he continued to counsel people in his home, which was near the beautiful greens of the Colonial Country Club—host to the famous Colonial Tournament on the PGA tour.

Many pastors, as did I, sought Dr. Kemp's sage advice in dealing with difficult counseling cases. "What can you say," I once asked, "when people are facing a situation so desperate that you are not sure that they can overcome it?"

Doctor Kemp smiled and replied with conviction, "You listen to them, and then offer them massive doses of hope. It is the best medicine this doctor can prescribe and is the essence of our faith."

Torch bearers are people whose journey brings us wisdom and wit, bravery and boldness. They persevere, overcome, and inspire others for living, loving, and journeying toward old age.

Reaching for the Stars: Ellen Ochoa, Ph.D.

Ellen Ochoa sets a living example for young Hispanic women, and for people everywhere, of what can result when you work to fulfill your dream. The first Hispanic woman in space, she has flown on four space shuttle missions aboard shuttles Discovery and Atlantis, serving as Payload Commander aboard the STS-66 Atlantis mission. She has logged over 978 hours in space and served as a mission specialist and a flight engineer. Earning her Master of Science and Doctor of Electrical Engineering degrees from Stanford University, Dr. Ochoa now serves as Deputy Director of the Johnson Space Center.[81]

Some people have a dream, but do nothing to turn their wish into reality. Some people reach for the stars and are willing to go the distance to soar among them. When they do, their dream becomes the star-dust of possibilities for others who need to know that they, too, have a chance.

Hill Country Sage: Oscar Glenn Sparks

Oscar Glenn Sparks sat in a chair across from me during a visit to his home. This eighty-nine-year-old husband and father lived alone in the Texas hill country. The visit also brought to mind the fond memory of my young sons' smiles of delight as they gave chase to goats that he kept behind his rural rock house. Glenn encouraged them with his laughter as they paid close attention to a wobbly newborn kid among the herd, knowing that the mother might display her displeasure and chase them out of the yard. Now, summoned to his home many years after that happy day, I sat knee-to-knee with him. I was aware of the gentle hum of a motor from a small device by his chair with the occasional puffing sound of pressurized air. It was an oxygen generator pumping the life-sustaining gas into his nostrils by way of clear-green plastic tubing. It was January 2006, and he was entering hospice care for end-stage chronic occlusive pulmonary disease. His wife was in a nursing facility with Alzheimer's Syndrome and he knew that his journey was winding down.

He looked into my eyes and profoundly declared to me a truth of human experience that we often do not put into words. He said, "You get to a place in your life where the days are not as bright, and you know that the days ahead are fewer than the ones behind you. You then reach back and pluck a memory from the past that you can hold onto and that brings you a smile, and that's what you take with you. You and your family are that kind of memory to me."

Glenn Sparks was more than a Hill Country goat rancher. He had served his country with honor in World War II, earning the Silver Star and a Purple Heart as a soldier with the 636th Tank Destroyer Battalion. After the war, he would spend the next forty-four years with the Southland Corporation in Dallas before retiring to the rural life he had known as a boy. His gruff exterior—sometimes cynical and sarcastic—gave way to a tender heart and a generous soul. He was a grandfather and great-grandfather who complained that he didn't especially like kids, and then donated a large sum of money needed for a playground at his church's preschool.

Some people make the world better by simply living in it. They press forward, keep faith, bear courage, offer loyalty, give devotion, and hide their vulnerability from all but those who care to find it. My life, and the life of my sons, is richer because of a Hill Country goat rancher with a soft-spot for preacher's kids and a wisdom that understands why relationships really matter.

Admirable Athlete and Humble Human: Michelle Wie

Michelle Wie was named by *Time Magazine* as one of one hundred people who have shaped our world. A Hawaii-born Korean-American athlete, Wie has overcome the odds to become a respected professional golfer. At age ten, she was the youngest player ever to qualify for the Women's U.S. Amateur Public Links Championship, a record unbroken for eight years until another ten-year-old Hawaiian accomplished the same feat. She broke many age records, being the youngest person to make the cut of an LPGA event, and the youngest person ever to win a USGA event.

Ms. Wie's generosity was clearly evident when she made a commitment of half a million dollars for Hurricane Katrina relief efforts at the same time that she turned professional, signing corporate sponsor contracts worth millions. Her hard work, professionalism, generosity, and outstanding character make her a torch bearer for professionals and amateurs, young and old, athlete and spectator[82].

Poet Laureate for Presidents and Everyday People: Maya Angelou

Maya Angelou rose out of poverty, abuse, and dire circumstances to become a renowned and respected poet and sage. Sharing her poem, "Morning," at the inauguration of President William Jefferson Clinton, and numerous appearances on the *Oprah Winfrey Show*, put her amazing talent, singular perspective, and vital wisdom on the national stage. Her poetry touches mind, emotion, and soul because it comes from the heart of one who knows the trials of life's journey and who has demonstrated the ability to transcend the tragedies that can befall us.

Ms. Angelou lives with the character that comes from one who holds deep convictions. Hers are convictions that hold belief in hope and possibility, with highest regard for learning, diligence, perseverance, equality, justice, truth, kindness, peace, love, and redemption.

A Zest for Life and Relationships: Kris Wheeler

Kris Wheeler was a wife and mother, office manager for a busy pediatrician, and "team mom" to whatever teenager needed her encouragement. She was also a woman who fought a brave battle with breast cancer. You will not see a marathon or research center named for her, but Kris represents countless women in this world whose strength in the face of adversity has been a source of strength for others.

Among her many pursuits, Kris loved to shop, and her favorite department store was Nordstrom. Growing up near the original Nordstrom store in Seattle, it became a custom, begun by her mother, for sisters and girlfriends, mothers and daughters, to enjoy a Saturday of shopping and swapping stories and laughter. This also led to one unique last request that Kris made of her husband, Wes.

On his way to Whidbey Island, Washington, and Kris's graveside funeral service, Wes stopped by the original Nordstrom store. The clerk with whom he spoke did not ask why, but simply fulfilled the request that he made of her through eyes filled with tears. Returning to his car, in the seat beside him was a container holding Kris ashes. She had desired cremation as the final disposition of her body.

When I stood at her grave in a small rural cemetery on Whidbey Island, Washington, it was not a casket or marble container that held her ashes. By her request, which Wes fulfilled, her remains where interred in a silver Nordstrom box swathed in a bright pink ribbon. It was one final tribute to her laughter and zest for life in all its joy.

Physicians, Pioneers, and Community Builders: Ed and Minnie Lee Lancaster

Doctors Ed and Minnie Lee Lancaster were quite a team. They graduated medical school and set up their practice in the small community of Grapevine, near Dallas, Texas. Minnie Lee was the first physician in Texas to give birth while in medical school, as female physicians were still a rarity. They raised their own family, and delivered countless babies to the families of that burgeoning community.

They became trusted family physicians in a town without a hospital, so they established one. Minnie Lee, the daughter of Methodist missionary parents, supported church and charity work in their city and made certain that a chapel was included in the plans as the hospital expanded. As a young man, just out of college, it was my privilege to work alongside them as an EMT in the busy emergency room of what was then Grapevine Memorial Hospital. It was Dr. Minnie Lee who helped me to explore my vocational calling beyond medicine to ministry, writing and counseling. It was during those years that Baylor Medical Center acquired the hospital and expanded its facilities and capabilities to serve the exploding population and development of the area.

They helped to build the community, and just before Minnie Lee's death, they gave a multi-million dollar gift for a multi-story patient tower at what had once been only a small, community hospital. Now, the tower bears their name. It is a visible presence of the regional medical center off Lancaster Drive that had its humble beginnings from two faithful physicians—a husband and wife team who lived lives of faith and devotion, building a community of healing while giving themselves away.

Generous Octogenarian: James R. Emanuel

I already began to tell the story of James Emanuel in the previous section, "Maintaining a Grasp of Stewardship." He was the gentleman who greeted each new day with excitement and a smile. He chose to take life for what it was as it came along, rather than having mountaintop expectations and dwelling too much on the past or the future (though he could tell a good story of days-gone-by!). His gratitude for life overflowed in a wise and generous stewardship of life, such that he made a financial fortune through diligence, thrift, and generosity.

He owned a lumberyard and hardware store in a small town and was generous with his customers. There was a man who built houses and who owed him a large sum of money. He had extended to this man a great deal of credit with the hope that the builder would sell the houses and then repay the debt he owed. Unfortunately, sales were down and the man could not afford to pay. Rather than undertake legal proceedings, he asked him what he had of value. The builder offered him some property which, at the time, was not of much value. It was on sloping land of rugged terrain that would be difficult to build upon, and there were no utilities nearby. The land did, however, overlook a nearby lake and so the vistas were beautiful. My friend accepted the offer of his customer in exchange for his debt. Years later, the seemingly worthless land became a much sought-after lakeside development with expensive homes built on very expensive lots. Out of his graciousness and generosity came a fortune and blessing. Before his death, James had given away millions of dollars in support of churches, colleges, seminaries, and orphanages. He helped to establish several new churches and supported Christian missionaries and international hunger relief programs. From his perspective, it was all just another day at the hardware store!

A Bright Spot in Anyone's Day: Grace Renick

Grace Renick is a source of joy that can brighten anyone's day by just being around them. She is the eternal optimist, life enthusiast, and spiritual oak who characterizes the best of Christian discipleship. Grace has been a part of Christ's holy church for a very long time and she has seen her share of ministers.

Grace said something to me that spoke volumes of her gracious faith and attitude. She said, "I have known many preachers in my lifetime, but I have never had a pastor who I didn't love." I have known some of the pastor's whom Grace has known, which is why her comment took me by surprise! Some were not the best of preachers. Some did not possess the most amiable personality. Some were neither winsome, nor witty, nor necessarily wise. Grace, on the other hand, is most all of those things and also bears the marvelous quality that her name implies—gracious. She models the value of believing in someone, desiring the best for them, and seeing the best in them. She is a faithful saint who supports God's servants and all God's children with her loving spirit and faithful presence.

Grace has the aches and pains that come with her advanced years. Her gait is not as stable, but her eyes still twinkle and her smile is memorable. A widow for decades, she could bemoan her losses or the passing of time, but she chooses to focus on the joy of living and the gift of loving. She is one of my favorite torch bearers, and I am blessed because, as her young pastor, she believed in me.

A Peace-Making Soldier: Colonel (Retired) George E. Bowers

Colonel (Retired) George E. Bowers is a family man and soldier. He has the heart of an explorer and the soul of a poet. As commanding officer of U.S. Army Camp Eagle during the Bosnian conflict, his mission was to keep the peace in a bitterly hostile environment while also protecting his troops. There was ethnic and religious tension, armed conflict, hazardous mines, and a desperate civilian population whose lives and economy had been decimated by war.

He spent time getting to know the people of the area he was protecting. He worked with the mayor of the nearby village and arranged for school supplies for the children and aid for families. It brought tears to his eyes to see the desperate plight of the people whose lives were made havoc by war, but whose spirits were indomitable. There was the man who had lost his house and his business, but he smiled back to Colonel Bowers and said with proud gratitude, "Thank God, I still have my family!"

Colonel Bowers missed his family. His wife, Susan, and children George, Jr., and Sarah, kept their own vigil and duties back home. Such is the life of a soldier's family. Such is the life of a professional soldier. Still, his focus was the safety and morale of his troops and the completion of his mission. He nurtured his spirit with daily prayer and devotional reading, and modeled for the troops the importance of care for body, mind, and spirit. He, as did they, wanted to return to the warmer and more hospitable climate of home, but loyalty and service kept them at their duty station.

Colonel Bowers is a man whose life embodies the army values of loyalty, duty, respect, selfless service, honor, integrity, and personal courage. He bears witness to these not only for the sake of his family and his country, but also for the sake of a grander good: peace for the human race.

Passing the Torch

These torch bearers of our life often kept their torch quietly hidden. We may not have known the hell that they had endured, the secrets that they had kept, or the chains of a troubled past that weighed them down. These truths, all the more, help us to appreciate their love, their sacrifice, and their devotion to us—even when it was expressed in ways that perhaps we didn't appreciate until much later.

There is a unique emptiness when such a torch goes out. Or does it? The torch continues in our memories and our lives. The torch is passed to us or others. Torches extinguished can be torches relit, and their flame can glow brighter than ever before.

The emptiness comes from the absence of one whom we loved, with whom we shared life, and from whom we received life. The gifts and legacy left behind continue as a positive reminder of their very best qualities and their precious contribution to the future. May we take with us the precious memories and sacred moments of such relationships. These need never die as long as memory lingers and gratitude grows.

With the help of God, may we look around us and open our

eyes to torch bearers in our life. They are there to offer us an icon of living and a leader to follow. What a gift we can give by valuing them in their lifetime. They also offer us the gift of their torch, for it lights the path that we have yet to journey. Perhaps their light might lead us to a new awareness of aging as a new horizon, and we are to be torch bearers that lead the march over the hill to tomorrow.

Aging as a New Horizon

When faculties and abilities diminish, it is hard to view aging so positively. It may even seem absurd to be celebrating something that ultimately leads to the end of our mortal journey. Therein is the rub: the *journey* is what life is about. Even the process of age-related changes can bring new horizons and open doors to other opportunities, relationships, experiences, hobbies, interests, and joys that we have yet to fully experience or explore.

For some, it is seeing the efforts of your labor bear much fruit as businesses and families prosper and grow. My father, at age eighty-five, celebrated his birthday with laughter and joy as he realized the many lives brought forth through his union with mother. His grandchildren and great-grandchildren are a source of joy and blessing that youth cannot comprehend nor possess. Only the perspective gained through growing older brings such joy.

In the motion picture, *The Guardian*, screenwriter Ron Brinkerhoff develops a wise and earthy character named Maggie McGlone, played by actress Bonnie Bramlett. She is the proprietor of "Maggie's Bar" in Kodiak, Alaska, a local "watering hole" and dance hall frequented by members of the Coast Guard, whose heroism is the subject of the film. She is talking late one night with Master Chief Ben Randall, played by Kevin Costner. He is a middle-aged, Coast Guard rescue swimmer who has sacrificed his marriage and his health for his career, and is unwilling to accept this reality as retirement closes in. Costner's character asks Maggie, "When did we get old?" She wisely and wryly replies:

> I don't mind [getting old]. If my muscles ache it's because I've used them. If it's hard for me to walk up those stairs it's because I've walked up them every night to lie next to a man who loved me. I've got a few wrinkles, but I've laid under thousands of skies on sunny days.... Getting old ain't bad; getting old—that's earned!"[83]

The world needs characters like Maggie McGlone to help us overcome our resistance to growing older. Such people are bridges, laying down their wisdom, experience, and positive life-perspective so that we can span the gap from youth to older adulthood without fear of what lies in-between. It is our resistance to growing older that sours the process and poisons our spirits, keeping us from enjoying the trek.

Successful and retired CEO's, authors, educators, parents, and grandparents are a precious resource to help others build a bridge over obstacles that they have already overcome. Such experience is invaluable to life, and is why the respect of elders is a significant teaching in most every culture. It has been said that how a society treats its most vulnerable citizens is a reflection of that culture's true values. Too many children live in poverty or without competent, caring parents to raise them. Too many older adults have inadequate access to sorely needed resources to assure their physical and emotional health and well-being. For us all to grow older without fear, we must also address issues of adequate resources for every person on the planet, and do so on an individual, neighborhood, community, municipal, county, state, national, and international level.

Look around where you live and see what needs to be done. Are there senior adults in your block or neighborhood who have no one to look after them? Are there older adults who do not have access to, or know how to gain access to, social services that would help them to age with grace instead of worry? What will you do about it? What if you were that adult? What would you want someone else to do for you?

If you are a retired executive, manager, business owner, professional, politician, or other leader, your new horizon can be to experience the fulfillment of sacrificial service by using your retirement "freedom" in service to others. Your life experience and professional expertise can be formidable tools to challenge political and social complacency. Use the power of your maturity to lead others who do not have your skills and network to resolve social issues for young and old. Be the voice for change on behalf of those who can only whisper in a world of selfish noise. Break through the wall of the status quo so that no one need grow up—or grow old—in a society where economics and misplaced priorities limit the possibility of success, health, and fulfillment for everyone.

Working for change begins at home. If you have children, have you spoken with them about their role as a caregiver to you as you grow older? How do you model for them the role of being a responsible caregiver to an older adult? If you do not have aging parents, you may consider "adopting" some through your area's Agency on Aging or a local senior care center. Leading by example is the best lesson of all.

To conclude this chapter on "Torch Bearers," I leave you

with the wisdom, hope, and blessing of this excerpt from the poem, "Sometimes:"

"Sometimes our best efforts do not go
amiss; sometimes we do as we meant to.
The sun will sometimes melt a field of sorrow
that seemed hard frozen: may it happen for you."[84]

For Reflection

1. Who has been a torchbearer in your life? What lesson did you learn or where were you led by their experience or example?

2. How might aging be a "new horizon" for your life? What attitude or action might you be called to take that would create your own "new horizon"?

3. Consider this thought: Changing jobs or changing careers is often not the answer. The solution may lie in changing yourself. How has failure to change impacted your life?

MAKING PEACE

Being at Peace with Life and All Its Changes

"Each morning I ask Melba how she's doing. 'I'm still kickin,'" she responds. Then I say, 'How high?'"
—Missy Buchanan[85]

"Lord, help me to remember that nothing is going to happen to me today that You and I together can't handle."
—An old preacher's greeting to each new day

"Things are exactly as they should be. If they were not, they'd be different!"
—Maxie C. Maultsby, Jr. M.D.

Working to Make it Happen

How we cope with aging is integral to how we face life. Our perspective defines us as individuals and how comfortable we are in our own skin. Our attitude reflects our values, beliefs, spirituality, economy, ego, empathy, priorities, and anxiety. Stereotypes, myths, misperceptions, fears, and misinformation all color our views on aging.

When we are intentional about what we want in life; we

work to make it happen. If we want to lose ten pounds, we make a plan and follow a plan to make it happen. If we want to compete in a 10K fun-run for a worthy charity, we train and workout to get in shape for the event. If we want to purchase our own home, we plan wisely, work diligently, save frugally, and make financial sacrifices for our dream to become a reality. If we want to live our life as best we can, to enjoy the journey and cherish the good times, we need to stop and examine our values, choices, hopes, and fears.

You are worth the effort it takes to make your life more mean-ingful. Your relationships will be more joyful, and your anxiety will be less troubling, when you address how you wish to live and what you want to do with your life. It is not too late to make some wise changes and choices. Every day is valuable.

Whether you have many days ahead of you or more days behind you, today is a day worth making better and more blessed. Embrace it, with all of its imperfections and disappointments, and know that life itself is a gift. Celebrate that gift by offering your love to someone else today, and remember God's three most precious gifts to us: life, love, and relationship. We are meant to be in relationship with each other and with God, without which both life and love are meaningless. Apart from relationship, life is merely isolation and love serves no purpose. I remind us once more that this is not an intention that all must be married; how-ever, committed relationships are crucial for family and children to exist in stability, security, and peace.

The Gifts of Mortality and Spirituality

Perhaps the best approach to aging is to remind ourselves of our own mortality and to use that reality to embrace life more fully.

When we do, we develop greater appreciation for relationships that give meaning to life, and the gifts that we each can offer to make life even richer and more blessed for all. It is arrogant and self-deceptive to deny or ignore that we will die one day.

We continue to act like the ancient societies, our ancestral cultures, who were unwilling to accept that mortality is something to be embraced rather than a reality to be feared. Just as they created so many gods and goddesses whose properties they thought might assuage the consequences of mortality, we make a gods of science, cosmetology, pharmacology, money and material things and then expect them to rescue us from the natural course of human experience. Mortality is our created nature. Whether you define it through means of science or religion (or bridge the two as did Teilhard de Chardin), our mortality—along with our character, actions, and spirituality—defines us. Aging is a part of our story and as such is a means of seeing our life in stages. These stages help us to better appreciate and value the time we share along the trek. Furthermore, growing older and our mortality help us to better cherish the relationships that we have with friends and loved ones. Aging is actually one means of grasping what is truly sacred: life!

It is our very nature to seek transcendence because of our need for relationship with the Divine. Though some individuals scoff at the spiritual, some seek God out of fear, and some religions engender the fear of damnation. Aging is more about maturing than decaying; aging is more about living than dying. Maturing is about developing as spiritual and enlightened people in spite of, or with the benefit of, an aging mortal body that holds an eternal and divine soul and a marvelous creative spirit. Our inner gifts, that part of us which others may not appreciate by merely gazing upon our outward appearance, can produce, create, inspire, build, comfort, and bring change to the world around us. We cannot become spiritually mature or whole in isolation, renunciation, or trepidation. Only in relationship, acceptance, and faith can we move toward being spiritually whole and embrace our physical journey and its inevitable changes with wonder and delight.

Though religion—a word whose etymology from one ancient Latin root meant "constraint"—has too often led to unconstrained and wasted effort fueling destructive diatribe, doctrinal war, and human tragedy, the true message and loving nature of the Creator God cannot be completely obscured or stifled for those who seek it. It is a truth that is vital to all who take this journey of life, and is a wonderful and refreshing truth that brings solace and calm to the human experience. It is the message that, accepted by faith, life is not ultimately about fear but about the journey itself. The changes and stages of life are all a part of what it means to be human. Whatever your faith or spiritual perspective, it is worth considering how Jesus brought to the human experience a revelation of God's true character: one of never-ending love, immeasurable mercy, and unimaginable creativity. Jesus knew a great deal about facing a journey without fear.

Spirituality addresses aging in context of the finite and the infinite: the mortal and the eternal. Spirituality is a vital resource for and cannot be separated from successful aging. We find inspiration and wisdom from sacred writings and the teachings of sage and revered leaders of faith.

The Dalai Lama, spiritual leader of the Tibetan people, in his book, *Advice on Dying and Living a Better Life*, reminds readers of an important teaching of Buddha:

A place to stay untouched by death
Does not exist.
It does not exist in space, it does not exist in the ocean,
Nor if you stay in the middle of a mountain.[86]

The book of Ecclesiastes, found in the Hebrew Bible (the Old Testament), tells us:

> For everything there is a season, and a time for every matter under heaven:
> a time to be born, and a time to die;
> a time to plant, and a time to pluck up what is planted;
> a time to kill, and a time to heal;
> a time to break down, and a time to build up;
> a time to weep, and a time to laugh;
> a time to mourn, and a time to dance;
> a time to throw away stones, and a time to gather stones together;
> a time to embrace, and a time to refrain from embracing;
> a time to seek, and a time to lose;
> a time to keep, and a time to throw away;
> a time to tear, and a time to sew;
> a time to keep silence, and a time to speak;
> a time to love, and a time to hate;
> a time for war, and a time for peace.
>
> Ecclesiastes 3:2

The Qur'an, holy book of Islam, emphasizes the gentle respect that the aged are due in The Children of Israel:

> And your Lord has commanded that you shall not serve (any) but Him, and goodness to your parents. If either or both of them reach old age with you, say not to them (so much as) "Ugh" nor chide them, and speak to them a generous word. And make yourself submissively gentle to

them with compassion, and say: O my Lord! have compassion on them, as they brought me up (when I was) little.

Your Lord knows best what is in your minds; if you are good, then He is surely forgiving to those who turn (to Him) frequently. And give to the near of kin his due and (to) the needy and the wayfarer, and do not squander wastefully.[87]

As I write this, I see a chirping finch sitting on a patio chair outside my window. It is enjoying the breezy, cool day, and the warmth of the bright sunshine reflected off the wind-whipped waves of the lake. It is doing what it knows to do: find food and water, fly on the breeze, seek shelter from the weather, interact with other birds, watch for predators, and enjoy living. There is no worry about growing older, though its lifespan is a fraction of mine.

I am reminded of Jesus' words from the Gospel of Matthew:

Therefore, I tell you, do not worry about your life, what you will eat or what you will drink, or about your body, what you will wear. Is not life more than food and the body more than clothing? Look at the birds of the air; they neither sow nor reap nor gather into barns, and yet your heavenly Father feeds them. Are you not of more value than they? And can any of you by worrying add a single hour to your span of life? And why do you worry about clothing? Consider the lilies of the field, how they grow; they neither toil nor spin yet I tell you, even Solomon [or to contemporize: Heidi Klum or Queen Elizabeth] in all his[/their] glory was not clothed like one of these. But if God so clothes the grass of the field, which is alive today and tomorrow is thrown into the oven, will he not much more clothe you—you of little faith? Therefore do not worry, saying 'What will we eat?' or 'What will we drink?' or 'What will we wear?'...indeed your heavenly Father knows that you need all these things. But strive first for the kingdom of God and his righteousness, and all these things will be given to you as well.

So do not worry about tomorrow, for tomorrow will bring worries of its own. Today's trouble is enough for today.

Matthew 6:25—31, 32b-34

Financial Peace

Fear of outliving one's income—lack of financial stability—is one of the five most significant fears mentioned earlier in this book from the survey on people's anxiety about aging. Quoting from Jesus' words encouraging followers not to worry may seem empty comfort to those evicted from their homes, bankrupt, and jobless during times of personal or national economic crisis. Yet there is great truth and promise to be found in these words.

Life is infinitely more than property, prosperity, and possessions. No external force can rob us of the true treasure of faith, love, hope, and inner peace if we choose to hold fast to these infinite and universal values. Both those who died and those who survived war, genocide, September 11, 2001, the Holocaust, and other great tragedies whose stories of perseverance are told, bear witness to this truth. When we hold fast amidst unrest and uncertainty, the anxiety of the unknown is placed in the larger perspective of hope.

While attending a Christmas service at a nearby church, I found both humor and profound wisdom in the words of an associate pastor of the congregation. She moved to the pulpit at the time of the offering. Before she said a prayer of blessing and thanksgiving for the gifts to be given, she made this statement: "If you view your life only from the perspective of the wealth that you own, remember that there are no pockets in a burial shroud and no hitch for a U-Haul on the back of a hearse!"

Financial peace is largely a matter of perspective and priority. Some of the poorest people whom I have encountered were more centered, deeply spiritual, and at peace with their life than many people whose bank accounts and lifestyle appear to be "comfortable."

One of the most sacred gifts which I have received was a crumpled dollar bill handed me by a frail, humble, Christian widow who resided in a nursing home. She reached for the pocket of her cable-knit sweater where she kept her meager monetary possessions, undid the large safety pin that held it shut, and handed me the dollar bill saying, "This is for my Lord!" I have never witnessed a more powerful expression of sacred stewardship, nor received any greater gift for Christ's Church, no matter how large the amount.

Financial peace is ultimately not about the balance of your bank account but your own balanced point of view of life, possessions, faith, and your future. We can make ourselves ill with worry about not having enough, and I personally know the anxiety of wondering if there will be enough money to provide for my family's needs in our monthly budget or if there will be more "month" than money. I say again, as a human family, we have all that we need to make this world work. There is enough to go around. When we spend wisely, save regularly, work diligently, live expectantly, give generously and seek the wisdom of those whose experience can help us produce and manage the resources we need, it is enough.

Can We Truly Be at Peace?

We can be at peace when we are anchored. On Christmas Day, 2008, I received an email from Charlie Ott, a college friend whose mother had just died. He spoke of being at her bedside at the moment of her passing from life, to death, to eternal life. There was the peace of knowing that her suffering was ended. There was also the reality of his now being an orphan, having already lost his father. We spoke of how both of us were orphans on that Christmas day, for each of us had said good-bye to the last of our parents.

There is emptiness in grief that no idealism can deny, and it would be naïve to think otherwise. Charlie and I are both orphans, though we have our own families and relationships as adults. We choose how we look upon what life's journey has brought. We walk a path comprised of both choices and irresistible, unstoppable outcomes. Acceptance of *how* life is, not necessarily *what* happens to us, is the key.

> *We can find greater peace when we accept that life is a journey of choices and chance, alternatives and inevitabilities, where we can change our own choices and perspectives but cannot control the choices of others or the immutable inevitabilities of life.*

It is this acceptance that can anchor us to the Truth that life is a gift of love from God who gives us hope and the opportunity to experience life for ourselves.

Life is not fatalism, nihilism, or perfectionism; but an opportunity and an adventure. I choose to make it an opportunity for good. I believe that we can make life better for ourselves and for others. I believe in possibility. I believe that love endures and overcomes. I believe that faith can transcend logic and despair. I believe that any religion more interested in rules than relationships is far-flung from the Divine. I believe that it is *how* we face life's inevitabilities and consequences that are more important than those outcomes. I believe that people whom culture may define as merely surviving may indeed be thriving far beyond what many hope to ever accomplish.

When I heard the testimony of two Holocaust survivors, the despairing conditions and seemingly hopeless circumstances that they experienced, I realized that these were individuals who thrived *while* they were in mid-plight because they did not give up! Society might not see it at the time, but there are people around us who are thriving by being courageous overcomers. Thriving is not merely to be successful or to have overcome, but to challenge overwhelming odds and persevere. Perseverance is, of itself, a means of thriving and living toward one's own best self and abilities.

We sometimes must remind ourselves that we are each on a journey that is interconnected. We need each other. We need to both receive and give God's love. We can live in peace when we step back and take stock of our life, then move forward along the path that takes us closer to God, toward self-acceptance and alongside those who need us. It is not merely the destination, but the *journey* that brings promise and fulfillment.

Life is about change, and that is inescapable. Transitions come, traditions change, and today will not last. All the more reason to live in the moment; cherish the present; and know that today's troubles need not define our entire journey. It is our challenge and our calling to claim hope as a gift for ourselves so that we can offer hope to those who only see life's despair.

Living in peace and believing in a good and loving God is more difficult when you are born into heartache. Deformities of body, dysfunction of family, victimization by the cruelty of others, and destruction by forces of nature that seem evil in their origin leave us questioning: "How can a God who is supposed to be loving and good allow this to happen?" Why does

God not end famine, calm the storm, and heal the sickened children? There are no easy answers, but I choose to believe that God's love of freedom that allows us to make choices on our journey also means that evil and heartache can occur, even when we do not bring it upon ourselves. Unknown or unpredictable actions of others may result in tragedy. The natural consequences of our mortality may lead to deformity and illness. Planetary forces and the randomness of nature may level cities. Were God to intervene in all of these, where would God's intervention end? Would we want the consequences of all our choices changed? What would happen to liberty and free will that give us the opportunity to face and incorporate the challenges of the journey as a part of our life? How can we appreciate the awesome, fulfilling, and holy experience of being *co-creators* with God if we are not given the privilege and opportunity to create, as well as the option to destroy or sit idle while the world desperately pleads us to act?

Given the nature of the universe and human existence, it is apparently not up to God to determine whether or not we live in peace; it is up to us. God has given us the opportunity to choose life or death, optimism or pessimism, hope or despair, love or hate, acceptance or denial, faith or disbelief, wholeness or brokenness, perseverance or surrender, and good or evil. God is neither an "absentee landlord" nor a cruel parent who watches helpless children struggle. No metaphor we may use can fully compare or describe the Divine nature and role in terms we can grasp. This I know for sure: God loves life so much that humanity is given birth as well as the opportunity to give birth to life, love, and hope when we appreciate the journey and job that is at hand. We were loved before we were conceived, redeemed before we were lost, and forgiven before we'd done wrong. Now it is up to us to live up to such a hallowed legacy. How will it be for you?

Let us continue, with renewed enthusiasm, the journey that has already been started. Ready. Set. *Go!*

For Reflection

1. Do you blame God for the evil of this world? Do you believe that God's choosing to give humankind free will also results in some randomness of life?

2. In 1 Corinthians, Chapter thirteen, the Apostle Paul wrote that love was greater than faith and hope. Do you agree with him? How are faith, hope, and love vital to living at peace with all of life's changes?

3. What is one thing that you will do to better face life and grow older without fear?

APPENDIX A

More Favorite Quotes and Poetry for Growing Older without Fear

Jenny kiss'd me when we met,
Jumping from the chair she sat in;
Time, you thief who love to get
Sweets into your list, put that in!
Say I'm weary, say I'm sad,
Say that health and wealth have missed me,
Say I'm growing old, but add,
Jenny kiss'd me.

—James Henry Leigh Hunt[88]

A nice example of someone combining exercise and learning was a man I met recently who was strapping himself into his hang-glider harness at age seventy-two. I must have looked a little surprised because he explained that this was something he had always wanted to do, but had not done before now because of family responsibilities. His children were fully independent and his wife had recently died, so he had just taken a course in flying a hand-glider and was about to go solo.

—Tom Kirkwood[89]

Now I am wandering about in "Dove's Lane" waiting, yet only three more weeks, to follow in the footprints of my Spouse, bound to Him by the Holy Vows of Poverty, Chastity, and Obedience.

—Sister Emma[90]

Young men and maidens,
old men and children.
Let them praise the name of the LORD,
for his name alone is exalted;
his splendor is above the earth and the heavens.

—Psalm 148:12–13

Another Definition of Aging:

Aging is the accumulation of changes in an organism or object over time. Aging in humans refers to a multidimensional process of physical, psychological, and social change. Some dimensions of aging grow and expand over time, while others decline. Reaction time, for example, may slow with age, while knowledge of world events and wisdom may expand. Research shows that even late in life potential exists for physical, mental, and social growth and development. Aging is an important part of all human societies reflecting the biological changes that occur, but also reflecting cultural and societal conventions.[91]

We could certainly slow the aging process down if it had to work its way through Congress.

—George H.W. Bush

On one of the written surveys about people's fears of growing older, a woman respondent, age sixty-five to sixty-nine, expressed this concern about heaven: "What will I look like when I get there? Will my loved ones recognize me?"

Another laughingly asked if I was interviewing any plastic surgeons for their point of view!

There's a lot of people in this world who spend so much time watching their health that they haven't time to enjoy it.

—Josh Billings

The only way to keep your health is to eat what you don't want, drink what you don't like, and do what you'd rather not.

—Mark Twain

Be careful about reading health books. You may die of a misprint.

—Mark Twain

I don't want to achieve immortality through my work…I want to achieve it through not dying.

—Woody Allen[92]

APPENDIX B

Assessing Dementia and Alzheimer's Disease

The Seven Warning Signs of Alzheimer's Disease (AD)

1. Asking the same question over and over again.

2. Repeating the same story, word for word, again and again.

3. Forgetting how to cook, how to make repairs or how to play cards: activities that were previously done with ease and regularity.

4. Losing one's ability to pay bills or balance one's checkbook.

5. Getting lost in familiar surroundings, or misplacing household objects.

6. Neglecting to bathe, or wearing the same clothes over and over again, while insisting that they have taken a bath or that their clothes are still clean.

7. Relying on someone else, such as a spouse, to make decisions or answer questions they previously would have handled themselves.[93]

Common Changes in Mild AD

- Loses spark or zest for life—does not start anything.

- Loses recent memory without a change in appearance or casual conversation.

- Loses judgment about money.

- Has difficulty with new learning and making new memories.

- Has trouble finding words—may substitute or make up words that sound like or mean something like the forgotten word.

- May stop talking to avoid making mistakes.

- Has shorter attention span and less motivation to stay with an activity.

- Easily loses way going to familiar places.

- Resists change or new things.

- Has trouble organizing and thinking logically.

- Asks repetitive questions.

- Withdraws, loses interest, is irritable, not as sensitive to others' feelings and/or uncharacteristically angry when frustrated or tired.

- Won't make decisions. For example, when asked what she wants to eat, says "I'll have what she is having."

- Takes longer to do routine chores and becomes upset if rushed or if something unexpected happens.

- Forgets to pay, pays too much, or forgets how to pay. May hand the checkout person a wallet instead of the correct amount of money.

- Forgets to eat, eats only one kind of food, or eats constantly.

- Loses or misplaces things by hiding them in odd places

or forgets where things go, such as putting clothes in the dishwasher.

- Constantly checks, searches, or hoards things of no value.

Common Changes in Moderate AD

- Changes in behavior, concern for appearance, hygiene, and sleep become more noticeable.

- Mixes up identity of people, such as thinking a son is a brother or that a wife is a stranger.

- Poor judgment creates safety issues when left alone—may wander and risk exposure, poisoning, falls, self-neglect, or exploitation.

- Has trouble recognizing familiar people and own objects; may take things that belong to others.

- Continuously repeats stories, favorite words, statements, or motions like tearing tissues.

- Has restless, repetitive movements in late afternoon or evening, such as pacing, trying doorknobs, fingering draperies.

- Cannot organize thoughts or follow logical explanations.

- Has trouble following written notes or completing tasks.

- Makes up stories to fill in gaps in memory. For example might say, "Mama will come for me when she gets off work."

- May be able to read, but cannot formulate the correct response to a written request.

- May accuse, threaten, curse, fidget, or behave inappropriately, such as kicking, hitting, biting, screaming, or grabbing.

- May become sloppy or forget manners.

- May see, hear, smell, or taste things that are not there.

- May accuse spouse of an affair or family members of stealing.

- Naps frequently or awakens at night believing it is time to go to work.

- Has more difficulty positioning the body to use the toilet or sit in a chair.

- May think mirror image is following him or television story is happening to her.

- Needs help finding the toilet, using the shower, remembering to drink, and dressing for the weather or occasion.

- Exhibits inappropriate sexual behavior, such as mistaking another individual for a spouse. Forgets what private behavior is, and may disrobe or masturbate in public.

Common Changes in Severe AD

- Doesn't recognize self or close family.

- Speaks in gibberish, is mute, or is difficult to understand.

- May refuse to eat, chokes, or forgets to swallow.

- May repetitively cry out, pat, or touch everything.

- Loses control of bowel and bladder.

- Loses weight and skin becomes thin and tears easily.

- May look uncomfortable or cry out when transferred or touched.

- Forgets how to walk or is too unsteady or weak to stand alone.

- May have seizures, frequent infections, falls.

- May groan, scream, or mumble loudly.

- Sleeps more.

- Needs total assistance for all activities of daily living. [95]

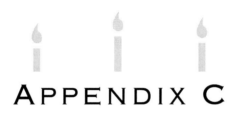

Appendix C

Resources for a Healthy Journey

Administration on Aging	www.aoa.gov
Alliance for Aging Research	www.agingresearch.org
Alzheimer's Association	www.alz.org
Alzheimer's Disease Education and Referral Center (NIA)	www.nia.nih.gov/alzheimers
Americans with Disabilities Online Resource	www.disabilityinfo.gov
AARP (formerly American Association of Retired Persons)	www.aarp.org/
Area Agency on Aging	(See your local listings)

Centers for Disease Control and Prevention	www.cdc.gov
Johns Hopkins Medical Letter: Health After 50	www.johnshopkinshealthalerts.com
Mayo Clinic: Tools for Healthier Lives	mayoclinic.com
National Association of Area Agencies on Aging	http://www.n4a.org/
National Cancer Institute	www.cancer.gov
National Institute on Aging	www.nia.nih.gov
National Institutes of Health	www.nih.gov
University of California at Berkeley Wellness Letter	http://wellnessletter.com/
U.S. Department of Health and Human Services	www.hhs.gov/aging/index.html

ENDNOTES

On The Run

1   David Carson (Director). (1994). S*tar Trek Generations* [Motion picture]. United States: Paramount Pictures.

2   Dr. Paul Kim, M.D., Gerontology, interview, January 29, 2006.

3   Tom Kirkwood, *"Time of Our Lives: The Science of Human Aging"* (Oxford: Oxford University Press, 1999), 10.

4   Jeffrey Scott Gall, PhD and Peggy Ann Szwbo, PhD, LCSW, RN/CCS, "Core Concepts: Psychosocial Aspects of Aging," *Clinical Geriatrics* 10, no. 5 (2002): 48–52.

5   Joan Goldwasser, "Aging Gracefully at Avon," *Kiplinger*, September 2004, 49; Matt Nesco, "GM's Market Value Half That of Avon," (CNBC.com, June 26, 2008), http://www.cnbc.com/id/25392542 (accessed Dec 31, 2008).

6   The American Society for Aesthetic Plastic Surgery, http://www.surgery.org/public/consumer/trends/cosmetic_procedures_in_2007 (accessed Feb 1, 2009)

7   Ibid.

8   Magali Rheault, "Facts and Figures," *Kiplinger*, September 2004, 22.

Naming Our Fear

9   Mike Stobbe, "Baby Boomers May Halt the Longevity Trend," *Fort Worth Star-Telegram*, December 9, 2005, 8A.

10   New Jersey Department of Health and Senior Services, http://www.state.nj.us/health/chs/19002000.html, (accessed February 29, 2008).

11   Ibid.

12   Stobbe, 8A.

13   2007 Human Development Report, United Nations Development Program. See also Anup Shah, "Poverty Facts and Stats," http://www.globalissues.org/TradeRelated/Facts.asp, (accessed April 27, 2008).

An American Perspective

14   Calum MacLeod. "A Glimpse of the Future: Robots Aid Japan's Elderly Residents." *USA Today*, November 5, 2009, http://www.usatoday.com/tech/news/robotics/2009–11–04-japan-robots_N.htm (accessed November 10, 2009).

15   Jeffrey Scott Gall, PhD and Peggy Ann Szwbo, PhD, LCSW, RN/CCS, "Core Concepts: Psychosocial Aspects of Aging," *Clinical Geriatrics* 10, no. 5 (2002): 48–52.

Taking A Deep Breath

16   Rob Reiner (Director). (2005). *Rumor Has It* [Motion picture]. United States: Warner Brothers Studios.

17   B. Glenn Wilkerson, Ron Lorimar, "The New Research Linking Unconditional Love with Self-Esteem and a Positive Self-Concept (1994 Study)," *ARK (Adults Relating to Kids)Programs*

Annual Report 2009, *University of Texas School of Public Health (Houston)*, (2009), Attachment A.

18 Eckhart Tolle, *A New Earth:Awakening to Your Life's Purpose* (New York: Plume, 2006), 139.

19 Life Without Limbs: Nick Vujicic, www.lifewithoutlimbs.org, (accessed September 10, 2009).

20 Jackson, Thomas. (Ed.). (1872) . *"A Plain Account of Christian Perfection,"* The Works of John Wesley (Ada,MI: Baker Books, 1996) Vol. 11, 383–385.

21 Reuben Job. *Three Simple Rules: A Wesleyan Way of Living* (Nashville: Abingdon Press, 2007).

22 Genesis 2:18

23 Matthew 19:24

24 U.S. Bureau of Labor Statistics, "Economic News Release, Table 2: Volunteers by Annual Hours of Volunteer Activities and Selected Characteristics," September 2007; http://www.bls.gov/news.release/volun.to2.htm (accessed July 29, 2008).

25 "Life Expectancy Reaches All-Time High in U.S.," Associated Press, August 19, 2009 (accessed August 19, 2009).

26 Vanessa Gisquet, "Ten Ways to Live Longer" *Forbes*, March 2, 2005, http://*Forbes*.com/ (accessed March 6, 2005).

27 "Adult Ministry Leaders Broaden Generational Understanding," United Methodist News Service, March 2, 2004 (accessed March 10, 2004).

A Fresh Perspective

28 Vanessa Gisquet, "Ten Ways to Live Longer" *Forbes*, March 2, 2005, http://*Forbes*.com/ (accessed March 6, 2005).

29 Gisquet. "Ten Ways to Live Longer."

30 Bob Arnot, M.D., "Ask Dr. Bob," *Men's Journal*, September 2008, 103.

31 Emily Dickinson, "Emily Dickinson, Number 1392," *Annabelle's Quotation Guide*, http://www.annabelle.net/ (accessed April 2, 2008).

32 Emily Dickinson, "Life Sonnet XXXII" in *The Collected Poems of Emily Dickinson*, ed. Martha Dickinson Bianchi (New York: Barnes & Noble Books, 1993), 19.

33 The Quotations Page, Robin Williams, U.S. Actor & Comedian (1951—), http://www.quotationspage.com/quote/36482.html (accessed August 2, 2008).

34 Norman Cousins, *Anatomy of an Illness as Perceived by the Patient* (Toronto: Bantam, 1981).

35 Society for Neuroscience, Brain Briefing, December 2001, "Humor, Laughter and the Brain," http://www.sfn.org/index. cfm?pagename=brainBriefings_humorLaughterAnd TheBrain (accessed August 3, 2008).

36 Society for Neuroscience, Brain Briefing, December 2001.

37 Sam Knight and Agencies, "Prayer Does Not Heal the Sick, Study Finds," *Times Online*, March 31, 2006, http://www.timesonline. co.uk/article/0,,11069–2112892,00.html (accessed July 25, 2008).

38 Wikiquote, "*Pierre Teilhard de Chardin*," http://en.wikiquote.org/ wiki/Pierre_Teilhard_de_ Chardin (accessed August 1, 2008).

39 *Book of Common* Prayer, "Burial Rite 1" (New York: Oxford University Press,1979), 485.

40 Norman Cousins, http://www.quoteworld.org/quotes/3224 (accessed October 12, 2008).

Making a Plan

41 James Brady. *"In Step With Ben Kingsley,"* Parade, June 22, 2008, 22.

42 Tony Care, "Chosen One," CBC Sports, Canada, August 1, 2008, http://www.cbc.ca/olympics/olympians/story/2008/07/31/f-olympics-feature-phelps.html (accessed August 27, 2008).

43 Gale Berkowitz, "UCLA Study on Friendship Among Women." (2002) http://www.scribd.com/doc/16043143/Ucla-Study-on-Friendship-Among-Women; and Taylor, S. E., Klein, L. C., Lewis, B. P., Gruenewald, T. L., Gurung, R. A. R, & Updegraff, J. A. Biobehavioral responses to stress in females: Tend-and-befriend, not fight-or-flight. *Psychological Review,* 107(3), (2000): 411–429 (accessed Jan 20, 2006).

Looking Over The Hill

44 Alzheimer's Disease Education and Referral Center, National Institute on Aging http://www.alzheimers.org/generalinfo.htm (accessed July 24, 2005).

45 Dr. Isadore Rosenfeld, "What You Need to Know Now," *Parade,* January 15, 2006, 6–7.

46 Alzheimer's Disease Education and Referral Center, National Institute on Aging, http://www.alzheimers.org/generalinfo.htm (accessed July 24, 2005).

47 Paul Kim, M.D., interview, January 29, 2006; and Depression-Guide.com, http://www.depression-guide.com/mini-mental-state-examination.htm (accessed, December 21, 2008).

48 Andrew Pollack, "Gene Therapy May Slow Alzheimer's," The New York Times, April 25, 2005. (See also, Nature Medicine,

online publication, www.nature.com/nm for a published paper on the trial.)

49 At the time of this interview, legislation to provide parity of insurance coverage for mental health was being drafted and debated by the U.S. Congress.

50 D.M. Parker, "Georgia's Cancer Awareness and Education Campaign: Combining Public Health Models and Private Sector Communications Strategies," Prevention of Chronic Diseases [serial online], Vol 1: No. 3, July 2004, http://www.cdc.gov/pcd/issues/2004/jul/04_0030.htm (accessed July 14, 2005).

51 National Cancer Institute, "A Snapshot of Prostate Cancer," http://planning.cancer.gov/disease/Prostate-Snapshot.pdf (accessed January 26, 2006).

52 Testicular Cancer Resource Center, http://tcrc.acor.org/tcprimer.html (accessed January 26, 2006).

53 Miranda Hitti, WebMD Medical News, March 2, 2005.

54 Multiple Sources: U.S. Dept. of Health and Human Services - Centers for Disease Control, National Immunization Program, Adult Immunization Schedule, http://www.cdc.gov/nip/recs/adult-schedule.htm (accessed. August 1, 2009); and General Board of Pension and Health Benefits-UMC, Personal Health Screening Guidelines, January 2006; and MayoClinic.com, "Health Screening Guidelines," http://www.mayoclinic.com/health/health-screening/W000112 (accessed January 26, 2009).

55 Dr. Steven Lamm, *The Hardness Factor: How to Achieve Your Best Health and Sexual Fitness at Any Age*, as quoted in *Newsweek* , May 30, 2005, 76.

Checking Out The Wildflowers

56 University of California—San Francisco School of Medicine, Osher Center for Integrative Medicine, *Integrative Medicine*. August 29, 2007, http://www.osher.ucsf.edu/About/Integrative Medicine.aspx (accessed October 12, 2008).

57 Vicki Johnson, MS, RYT, "Louise Gartner, Yoga Pioneer of Dallas," *Holistic Networker*, Spring 2005, 39.

58 *Yoga* Journal, February 2005, as quoted by Colleen Long, "Yoga For All Sizes," *The Dallas Morning News*, June 14, 2005, 5E.

59 Colleen Long, *The Dallas Morning News*, 5E.

60 G.C. de los Reyes, R.T. Koda, and E.J. Lien, "Alternative Medicine that Actually Works?," *Geriatrics and Aging*, Volume 4, No. 5, June/July 2001, p 9,30,31, www.geriatricsandaging.ca. (accessed June 15, 2005).

61 Julie Dergal, MSc., Paula A. Rochon, MD MPH, FRCPC, "What Physicians Should Know About Herbal Medicines: Potential Drug Interactions in Older People," *Geriatrics and Aging*, 4, no.5, (2001): 28, 29, www.geriatricsandaging.ca (accessed January 15, 2006).

62 Jessica Ryen Doyle, *Michael Phelps' 12,000 Calorie-a-Day Diet Not For Everyone*, Fox News, August 14, 2008, http://www.foxnews.com/story/0,2933,403803,00.html (accessed October 14, 2008).

63 U.S. Department of Health and Human Services and U.S. Department of Agriculture, *Dietary Guidelines for Americans*, http://www.mypyramid.gov/guidelines/index.html,   (accessed October 14, 2008).

64 Dr. Isadore Rosenfeld, "What You Need to Know Now," *Parade*, January 15, 2006, 7.

65 Rosenfeld, 7.

66 MayoClinic.com, "Health Screening Guidelines," http://www. mayoclinic.com/health/fish-oil/NS_patient-fishoil (accessed January 26, 2006).

67 Abdullah Fatteh, M.D., and Naaz Fatteh, M.D., "*Young At Any Age: Prescriptions for Longevity*" (Cambridge MA: Brookline Books, 2001), 25.

68 National Institutes of Health–Office of Dietary Supplements, *Dietary Supplement Fact Sheets*, *h*ttp://ods.od.nih.gov/Health_ Information/Information_About_Individual_Dietary_ Supplements.aspx (accessed October 11, 2008).

69 NIH-ODS, *Fact Sheet*.

Taking An Alternate Route

70 Gene Cohen, M.D., Ph.D., "The Myth of the Midlife Crisis," *Newsweek*, Vol. CXLVII No. 3, January 16, 2006, 82.

71 Via E-mail from John C. Pace, April 22, 2005.

72 Tom Kirkwood, "*Time of Our Lives*," 8.

73 Maddy Dychtwald, "Adult Ministries Institute 2004," San Francisco, *United Methodist News Service*, March 2, 2004.

74 TiVo is a registered trademark of TiVo, Inc.

75 "Goal 4: Reduce Child Mortality," worldbank.org, (accessed August 9, 2009)

76 Nothing But Nets Campaign, http://www.nothingbutnets.net/ (accessed May 1, 2009)

77 Dave Roever Ministries, http://www.daveroever.org/ (accessed January 20, 2006)

78 Gale Berkowitz, "UCLA Study on Friendship Among Women." (2002) http://www.scribd.com/doc/16043143/Ucla-Study-on-Friendship-Among-Women; and Taylor, S. E., Klein, L. C., Lewis, B. P., Gruenewald, T. L., Gurung, R. A. R, & Updegraff, J. A. Biobehavioral responses to stress in females: Tend-and-befriend, not fight-or-flight. *Psychological Review*, 107(3), (2000): 411–429 (accessed Jan 20, 2006).

79 Gale Berkowitz, "UCLA Study on Friendship Among Women," (2002).

Torch Bearers

80 "Willa Player, Pioneering College President," *United Methodist News Service*, September 12, 2003, http://archives.umc.org/umns/news_archive2003.asp?ptid=2&story=%7B0268A2C2–2BC4–4E39-A727–31653D40D539%7D&mid=2406 (accessed January 20, 2006).

81 National Aeronautics and Space Administration, *Ellen Ochoa Biographical Data*. January 2008, http://www.jsc.nasa.gov/Bios/htmlbios/ochoa.html (accessed December 7, 2008).

82 Bob Chaundy, Faces of the Week: Michelle Wie, *BBC News*, July 29, 2005, http://news.bbc.co.uk/2/hi/uk_news/magazine/4727895.stm (accessed Feb 1, 2008).

83 Andrew Davis (Director). (2006). *The Guardian* [Motion picture]. United States: Touchtone Pictures.

84 Sheenagh Pugh. "Sometimes." (Brigend, Wales:Seren Books) 1990.

Making Peace

85   Missy Buchanan, "Aging Well: 'I'm Just Here,'" *United Methodist Reporter*, July 16, 2008, http://www.umportal.org/main/article.asp?id=3803 (accessed July 18, 2008).

86   Dalai Lama, *Advice on Dying and Living a Better Life*, translated and ed. by Jeffrey Hopkins, PhD. (New York: Atria Books, 2002), 40.

87   The Qur'an, 17.23-.26.

Appendix A

88   James Henry Leigh Hunt, "Jenny Kissed Me." http://www.cs.rice.edu/~ssiyer/minstrels/poems/103.html (accessed August 25, 2009).

89   Tom Kirkwood, *"Time of Our Lives,"* 238.

90   David Snowdon,Ph.D., *"Aging with Grace"* (New York: Bantam Books, 2001) 101.

91   Wikipedia contributors, "Ageing," *Wikipedia, The Free Encyclopedia*, http://en.wikipedia.org/w/index.php?title=Ageing&oldid=310521516 (accessed August 28, 2009).

92   Woody Allen, "Wisdom Quotes:, http://www.wisdomquotes.com/001043.html (accessed July 15, 2008).

Appendix B

93   The Suncoast Gerontology Center, University of South Florida. Revised 9/01/99, posted via Alzheimer's Disease Education and Referral Center, National Institute on Aging, http://www.alzheimers.org/pubs/sevensigns.htm (accessed January 20, 2006).

94 Lisa P. Gwyther, *Caring for People with Alzheimer's Disease: A Manual for Facility Staff,* 2nd ed., (Washington D.C.: American Health Care Association, 2001) http://www.alzheimers.org/pubs/stages.htm (accessed January 20, 2006).